"From the perspective of a family physician with obesity medicine training, Crowley's book is a remarkable blend of scientific rigor, clinical wisdom drawing from decades of experience, and holistic compassion that will enlighten and empower therapists who wants to help their clients understand and overcome their eating disorder."

Dr Nick Knear-Bell, MD, *American Board of Obesity Medicine Diplomate, NASM nutritionist*

"Eating disorders are among the most challenging and potentially lethal problems mental and behavioral health clinicians encounter. Beyond the need for scientifically grounded treatment, they also require a great deal of clinical artistry to succeed. This is why Bethany Crowley's fantastic book, is an absolute gem. In a wonderfully warm and inviting manner, Bethany weaves together the art and science of effective care for eating disorders. Indeed, she provides a template for a great deal of powerful, behavioral health care methods that easily transcends any single diagnosis or condition. I will happily recommend this fine book to my patients and colleagues alike!"

Clifford N. Lazarus, PhD, *NJ licensed psychologist, co-founder & director,*
The Lazarus Institute for Multimodal Therapy

An Integrative Approach to Treating Eating Disorders

An Integrative Approach to Treating Eating Disorders walks therapists through how to effectively resolve the most common yet nuanced struggles that clients with disordered eating face on a daily basis.

This straightforward workbook begins by demystifying the complexities and nuances of eating disorders. It then helps therapists understand the need for an integrative approach and walks them through how to assess a client's biological, psychological, social, and spiritual domains as they correlate with disordered eating behaviors and thoughts. This is accomplished with the BASIC I.D. assessment model and a multimodal therapy framework, both created by Dr Arnold Lazarus. Nine foundational skills are provided for clients to achieve lasting recovery and avoid the all-too-common relapse rate of eating disorders.

Each foundational skill is presented in its own chapter, complete with data, case vignettes, worksheets, and exercises developed over twenty years of research and client management. With this book, therapists both new and experienced will boost their confidence, gain practical tools, and bring more efficiency to their individual or group sessions.

Bethany C. Crowley, LMFT, CEDS, BCN is the founder and clinical director of The Journey Therapy, an intensive outpatient program for those with eating disorders. She is a certified eating disorders specialist with more than twenty years experience treating the struggles of food and body image through direct client care.

An Integrative Approach to Treating Eating Disorders

9 Foundational Skills for a Lasting Recovery

Bethany C. Crowley

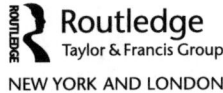
Routledge
Taylor & Francis Group

NEW YORK AND LONDON

Designed cover image: johnwoodcock © Getty Images

First published 2024
by Routledge
605 Third Avenue, New York, NY 10158

and by Routledge
4 Park Square, Milton Park, Abingdon, Oxon, OX14 4RN

Routledge is an imprint of the Taylor & Francis Group, an informa business

© 2024 Bethany C. Crowley

ISBN: 9781032651392 (hbk)
ISBN: 9781032635125 (pbk)
ISBN: 9781032651408 (ebk)

DOI: 10.4324/9781032651408

Typeset in Galliard
by Newgen Publishing UK

For my son Tyler,
"Do things close to your heart with passion and dedication."

Contents

Introduction

In my practice of over twenty years, I have worked with hundreds of individuals struggling with issues regarding food and body image. And while these people have certain qualities and traits that make them more vulnerable to developing an eating disorder, the complexities of the underlying issues combined with the uniqueness of their personal experiences make this disorder challenging to treat.

When relapse occurs, it's disheartening for those struggling and their families—and discouraging for the treatment team as well. Relapse can be an exasperating and repetitive process that causes individuals and providers to lose not only motivation but the optimism that lasting recovery from an eating disorder is possible.

For this reason, through working with this population for more than two decades, my focus has been on paying meticulous attention to my clients and fellow providers, both of whom have shared with me their challenges about their experiences with the eating disorder recovery process. As I carefully listened to their stories, I extracted several common themes around barriers to treatment and recovery. I made it my mission to eradicate these barriers and challenges—and that's when I identified the nine essential skills needed in building a foundation required for lasting eating disorder recovery. The mastery of these nine skills is consistently lacking when individuals relapse.

Clinicians and other professionals begin their work with questions similar to those of their clients. We are desperate for answers—and for effective practical strategies and solutions on what to do next.

- Where would I ...?
- What do I do if...?
- How do I work with...?
- When would I...?
- Who would...?

The answers to these important questions are the impetus for this book.

Fortunately, in the last decade, there are more resources available on the topic of disordered eating. This was not the case when I first started in this field. As a new therapist, I searched for an integrative book that used a biopsychosocial framework to help me to understand eating struggles (although I didn't exactly know that that's what I needed back then). I wanted a comprehensive guide that contained detailed nuances in order to gain a better understanding of eating struggles, that shed light on the underlying problems that fuel disordered eating, and that contained effective treatment plans for recovery. I often asked my clients what they felt they needed, but most did not know and were not able to articulate their needs—however, they could clearly describe their hardships with food and body image. I searched for a resource that provided techniques, strategies, tools, and effective practice worksheets that would aid in my client's treatment starting at intake through discharge.

Unfortunately, that book did not exist back then.

The Integrative, Biopsychosocial Framework Unique to this Book

Due to a lack of effective, comprehensive resources, I developed my own exercises and interventions to help my clients understand disordered eating concepts. They had a desire to know the "why" behind the tools that I created and used with them. In doing this, it became clear that when my clients could comprehend the reasoning behind

DOI: 10.4324/9781032651408-1

each skill, they immediately felt better, more integrated, and at ease. I felt that this insight was a significant component missing in resources for helping people recover from disordered eating.

Psychoeducation is an essential part of my method in treating eating disorders. Helping clients to understand how their thoughts, behaviors, feelings, and perceptions are connected to their eating struggles and body dissatisfaction has been a cornerstone to the effectiveness of my approach. For example, people who struggle with eating often have difficulties asking questions when things don't make sense (this can be due to their anxiety or a need for control). If they don't ask questions, how can they expect to get better? Thus, it's our job to help them gain clarity around their issues, so they can eventually ask the right questions—and then better follow and practice the skills needed for eating disorder recovery.

In addition to developing interventions, exercises, tools, and worksheets, I developed a comprehensive eating disorder recovery treatment guide. In my quest to find the ultimate eating disorder treatment book, I inadvertently ended up writing the book I had searched for over the course of my career. *An Integrative Approach to Treating Eating Disorders: 9 Foundational Skills for a Lasting Recovery* is an evidenced-based comprehensive treatment guide that gives a framework and method on how to treat arguably the most complex of disorders.

This ultimate integrative guide helps practitioners understand eating struggles from intake to discharge. It will help any clinician build confidence in having an effective plan to help their clients resolve their eating issues and allows therapists to utilize their own style and approach to help develop foundational skills, depending on their client's needs. This is a simple-to-follow book written as a clinician's companion—complete with valuable teaching tools designed to help you help your client cultivate the skills needed to build their foundation for a solid recovery.

How to Use This Book

The first chapter covers the principal elements for understanding often *misunderstood* eating disorders; it focuses on the complexities, issues, and challenges that make eating disorders tricky to treat. The second chapter introduces my method, including the steps needed to uncover the basis of your client's eating disorder. The underlying issues are then addressed in your therapy sessions.

The remaining chapters each tackle one of the nine foundational skills essential for eating disorder recovery. The foundational skills are used to manage the symptoms of your client's struggles with eating and are skills that your client hasn't yet developed but are needed in life and for their recovery. Each chapter offers background about why each skill is essential to recovery and how it is related to your client. You will learn how your client's eating struggles may worsen if the skill is not mastered. Each foundational skill comes with both clinician and client tools, exercises, and worksheets that can be used as interventions and homework for your treatment plan.

The chapters are presented in the order most beneficial for the clinician and most effective for your client. However, after conducting an assessment (such as if your client has had previous treatment), it's important to understand the stage your client is at by determining which of the foundational skills have been mastered and which need to be improved upon.

Your outcomes are measured by your client's ability to apply each of the foundational skills effectively and the improvement of their eating disorder. There are examples of a treatment plan, clinical note, and a discharge note in the epilogue.

In my experience, working with complications as they arise has been effective. Over time, the client learns how to deal with each symptom as it surfaces, allowing them to feel empowered rather than discouraged. As each issue is managed, they feel less overwhelmed and more effective in dealing with challenges. They learn effective tools that help them to separate, extract, and isolate certain symptoms so that they can practice working through each feature instead of trying to deal with all issues at once. This promotes self-efficacy, allowing them to feel that they can overcome and deal with highly emotional, uncomfortable situations.

It is important to note that while this method is effective, it is important to confirm that your client is at the appropriate level of care clinically. The method outlined in this book is most effective only after your client is medically stable and able to cognitively function. For example, if your client is restricting food and has been compromised medically and cognitively, they will not be able to retain any of this information. The priority in a case like this would be for them to receive inpatient medical attention where the priorities are for medical stability and refeeding. It is strongly recommended, if you are a newer clinician in this field, that you have clinical supervision by someone who specializes in disordered eating.

Effective Treatment Is Possible

According to the Eating Disorders Coalition, every sixty-two minutes at least one person dies of an eating disorder. Eating disorders are among the mental disorders with the highest mortality rates. If individuals do not receive effective treatment, it is literally life or death for them. In addition, eating disorders have a high relapse rate. According to the Eating Disorders Coalition, approximately 40 percent of all who seek treatment will relapse. These are staggering statistics. But with this book, you can help your client avoid being another victim.

Whether you are new to working with eating disorders, or have an interest in specializing in the field and are looking for resources to help in therapy sessions, or you are a veteran but still find yourself saying, "I wish I had better tools for my client!" this book can help. My hope is that this comprehensive guide will give you a streamlined method and plan to effectively help your clients achieve a solid recovery. Teaching my clients social-emotional skills to manage stressful life events has sustained their recoveries. The same can happen for your clients.

Part I

An Integrative Skills-Building Approach to Treating Eating Disorders

Chapter 1

The Misunderstood Eating Disorder

Eating disorders are arguably the most complex of all mental health disorders. Due to their nuanced nature, therapists often struggle with where to start. This struggle is so pervasive that it is the impetus for this book. How to go about treating your client is intimidating, but truthfully the whole treatment process can appear daunting. There are so many aspects that are intertwined, and everything can feel urgent because these features affect all areas of your client's life, physically, emotionally, cognitively, behaviorally, and spiritually. Sometimes, just hearing about all of the disordered eating behaviors that your client is engaging in and the intense emotions that they are experiencing can lead you to question your effectiveness as their therapist.

Fortunately, with the integrated, comprehensive biopsychosocial framework presented in this book, you'll learn where to start, how best to approach various scenarios, and determine what to do to treat your clients effectively.

Before we get into specifics, let's take a look at a case example Nicole, who we'll return to periodically throughout this chapter and Chapter 2.

Case Example: Nicole, 19

Nicole, 19, sought out therapy to deal with her anxiety and depression after the breakup of her two-year relationship. The first session:

Therapist: *"What brings you here today?"*

Nicole: *"I don't know. I called because I've been extremely sad and haven't been able to sleep. I cry all the time and can't relax. I feel like I'm in a daze and am not all there. I'm exhausted and have a headache. My chest hurts. I feel weak and sleepy, but still can't relax or sleep. The hardest part for me is when I doze off, I wake up with my heart pounding out of my chest and I remember that I don't have a boyfriend anymore, and this is a real nightmare, I'm alone. I have these bad thoughts about myself. I feel empty and scared and want to throw up. I went to see my family doctor and they sent me here. They said that they couldn't really help me, and that I probably just need to talk to someone."*

Therapist: *"Ok. Sounds like you're going through a lot right now. I'm glad that you're here."*

Nicole: *"I don't really want to be here, but I don't know what to do. I don't want to feel this badly anymore. I'm going through a lot. My boyfriend broke up with me after two years of being together. He just did it out of the blue. I didn't see it coming. I got fired from my job last week because I didn't call into work and just didn't show up. My boss doesn't exactly like me after that incident with my co-workers that I don't really want to go into right now. There was no way I could go to work. I was so sick and threw up all day. I was too embarrassed to see anyone or to bump into someone I know. I guess, it shouldn't be such a surprise that he broke with me. I knew when I first met him, I shouldn't trust him. I don't normally trust anyone, but I was stupid. I'm so stupid. Why was I so stupid to believe that someone would love me? It's just my own stupid fault. My parents tried to warn me, but I didn't listen. I don't necessarily want my mom's advice when I see how messed up she and my dad are. But I guess they're right, no 'good' guy will love someone like me. I just hoped that things could be different. I tried to imagine things could change. I guess, this just proves that things can't change. It'll always be bad."*

Therapist: *"Tell me more about this relationship."*

DOI: 10.4324/9781032651408-3

Nicole:	*"He just broke up with me. He said he just needed space to figure things out. I know it's because of me. I knew he really couldn't love me. I don't normally say this out loud to people I don't know but I know he didn't really love me because look at me. I'm not exactly his type."*
Therapist:	*"Tell me more."*
Nicole:	*"I'm bigger than the girls he usually dates. I knew he didn't want to be with me. I tried to save myself pain. I even made sure by asking him if he was sure he wanted to be with me. I'd point out other girls and tell him that he could be with them and wonder why he was with me. I was careful and he always told me he loves me, but now I know it's a lie. He's probably with someone else right now and happy. I feel sick. I feel really sick thinking about it."*
Therapist:	*"Sounds like you're experiencing a lot of uncomfortable feelings right now."*
Nicole:	*"Yes, and I have no one to talk to. I can't talk to my parents. And honestly, I don't really have the kind of friends I can talk to about this stuff. Plus, I don't even want to talk to anyone about this. I've been alone for the last few days. I feel sick. I have headaches and feel so weak."*
Therapist:	*"Tell me more about what you mean when you say, I feel sick."*
Nicole:	*"I literally feel physically sick, like I want to throw up. I've been throwing up and at least feel a little relief but then I feel so weak afterwards. I don't want to eat but I know I have to. But right now, I just can't eat. Part of me feels sick and full and don't want to eat and the other part of me feels like I don't deserve to eat at all. I don't know how you're going to help me. This all feels hopeless."*

Nicole has a lot going on! Understandably, therapists may feel discouraged and maybe even intimidated by this example. What's clear is that Nicole is growing through a breakup and experiencing interpersonal challenges in various relationships, including her perception about her nuclear family. But is Nicole's throwing up and loss of appetite a symptom of her relational issues or result of everything else? Some red flags that can indicate a possible eating disorder is her belief that she doesn't deserve to eat, throwing up, and body dissatisfaction. Yet it is difficult to have a clear diagnosis with the limited information. This is an example of why eating disorders are considered one of the most complicated disorders to treat, with discouraging relapse rates. We'll revisit Nicole's treatment scenario in Chapter 2, where you'll learn the most effective treatment process to approach this case.

What is an Eating Disorder?

Treating eating disorders is truly a specialized field and is an area that is rarely taught in academic programs. And when this subject matter is presented, it is usually a general overview about eating disorders that can be found in the DSM -5-TR and looks something like this:

Standardized Definition

Here's a summary of how the DSM -5-TR describes the following disorders:

The following eating disorders with the exception for Binge Eating Disorder (BED) share the characteristic of Body Dissatisfaction:

- Disturbance in the way in which one's body weight or shape is experienced, undue influence of body weight or shape on self-evaluation, or denial of the seriousness of the current low body weight.

Anorexia Nervosa, characterized by:

- Restriction of energy intake relative to requirements, leading to a significantly low body weight.
- Intense fear of gaining weight or becoming fat or persistent behavior that interferes with weight gain.

Bulimia Nervosa, characterized by:

- Recurrent episodes of binge eating within any two-hour period, an amount of food that is relatively larger than what most individuals would eat in a similar period of time within similar circumstances.
- A feeling that one cannot stop eating or control what or how much one is eating.

- Recurrent inappropriate compensatory behaviors in order to prevent weight gain include self-induced vomiting, misuse of laxatives, diuretics or other medications, and fasting and excessive exercise.
- The binge eating and inappropriate compensatory behaviors both occur on average at least once a week for three months.
- Self-evaluation is unduly influenced by body shape and weight.
- The disturbance does not occur exclusively during episodes of anorexia nervosa.

Binge Eating Disorder, recurrent episodes of binge eating.

1. An episode of binge eating is characterized by both: a) eating in a discrete period of time (for example, within any two-hour period), an amount of food that is definitely larger than most people who eat in a similar period of time under similar circumstances; b) a sense of lack of control overeating during the episode (for example, a feeling that one cannot stop eating or control what or how much one is eating).
2. The binge-eating episodes are associated with three (or more) of the following:

    - Eating much more rapidly than normal.
    - Eating until feeling uncomfortably full.
    - Eating large amounts of food when not feeling physically hungry.
    - Eating alone because of feeling embarrassed by how much one is eating.
    - Feeling disgusted with oneself, depressed, or very guilty afterwards.
    - Marked distress regarding binge eating is present.
    - The binge eating occurs, on average, at least once a week for three months.
    - The binge eating is not associated with the recurrent use of inappropriate compensatory behavior (for example, purging) and does not occur exclusively during the course of anorexia nervosa, bulimia nervosa, or avoidant/restrictive food intake disorder.

Some of the lesser-known disorders found in the DSM-5-TR include the following.

Other Specified Feeding Eating Disorders (OSFED) was previously known as Eating Disorder Not Otherwise Specified (EDNOS):

- Atypical Anorexia Nervosa: All criteria are met except despite significant weight loss, the individual's weight is within or above the normal range.
- Bulimia Nervosa (of low frequency and /or limited duration): All of the criteria for bulimia nervosa are met, except that the binge eating and inappropriate compensatory behavior occurs at a lower frequency and/or for less than three months.
- Purging Disorder: Recurrent purging behavior to influence weight or shape in the absence of binge eating.
- Night Eating Syndrome: Recurrent episodes of night eating. Eating after awakening from sleep, or by excessive food consumption after the evening meal. The behavior is not better explained by environmental influences or social norms. The behavior causes significant distress/impairment. The behavior is not better explained by another mental health disorder (e.g., BED).

These definitions are straightforward and clear. But the reality is that eating disorders are rarely that. They're not always overt or linear. They can morph from one to the other. They can be hidden or disguised as "healthy" eating. With such rigid definitions and limited information on treatment protocols, it is not surprising that most clinicians starting out who have never been supervised in a practicum setting such as an eating disorder treatment center or program have relatively little understanding of how to treat eating disorders and will have difficulty knowing where to start and should refer their client to someone who has relevant experience. And yet, even for those fortunate enough to have trained in an eating disorder treatment program, given the complexities of eating disorders it can still be challenging to find the most effective treatments with lasting results.

A More Nuanced Portrait of Eating Disorders

Due to the nature of eating disorders and how they manifest, change, and transform, it can be challenging to recognize when someone has issues with food or has an eating disorder. Therapists that are just starting to work with these individuals may have difficulty recognizing potential problems and their behaviors may not appear obvious.

The following chart is the result of decades of research and helping hundreds of clients and includes some of the more common as well as the subtler signs of an eating disorder. The more signs that individuals have, the stronger the indicator that they may be struggling with an eating disorder. In addition, some are more prevalent in certain disorders. Along with a detailed client intake and assessment, this list can help you to identify a general issue and offer insight into the nature of the disorder your client is dealing with.

Why Are Eating Disorders Complicated to Treat?

It is important to acknowledge that the lack of effective treatments and high numbers of relapse rates is due to the prevalence of people that struggle with this disorder (Sala et al. 2023). Eating disorders are a global issue among young people (Silén & Keski-Rahkonen 2022).

According to the Eating Disorder Hope website approximately 20 million females and 10 million males in the US alone has had a significant clinical eating disorder at some point in their life. Therefore, it is highly likely that someone will come to you seeking help for this problem. In addition, the mortality rate of eating disorders is one of the highest compared to any other disorder: 10% of those diagnosed with an eating disorder will die from it.

These stark statistics paint a dreary picture. If individuals do not get the help they need, these statistics will continue. So why is it so hard for us clinicians to treat those with eating problems? Why are there ineffective treatments and discouraging rates of relapse? Let's look at several reasons.

Treating Eating Disorders Requires Specialized Training

Understanding and treating eating disorders requires a diverse knowledge base, skill at clinical interventions and techniques, a clear methodology and process, and identified goals and outcomes. But graduate programs do not cover eating disorders in standard coursework. Therefore, clinicians interested in learning about how to treat eating disorders will need to seek out specialized trainings but it can be challenging to find this. Fortunately, more eating disorder training is now online, and most eating disorder treatment programs offer courses. However, some training may not be sufficient and ongoing training is necessary. If a therapist is just starting out, they will need to have clinical supervision.

Even with specialized training under one's belt, another barrier arises: putting together a proper care team. Due to the nature and complexities of eating disorders, it is essential that clients work with a physician, dietitian, *and* psychotherapist knowledgeable in treating eating disorders. In some rural areas, there is a shortage of these which can be challenging for a client—and for you.

When a client doesn't have access to professionals trained in eating disorder treatment, they are then faced with an adverse likelihood: *Well-meaning therapists can unintentionally give detrimental suggestions.*

A therapist's natural tendency is to want to help the client resolve their body image and food issues. But due to insufficient training their suggestions are often misguided—and can be harmful and even detrimental to clients. Here are real quotes from real clients who came to me after their treatment under other therapists seemed to be failing:

Therapist suggestion:	"My last therapist knew I was afraid to eat over 900 calories, so she told me to track and record my calories."
Why it is not helpful:	Individuals who struggle with eating are already hyper fixated on food, calories, weight, size etc. Having someone with an eating disorder track calories actually fuels their eating disorder by encouraging a focus on calories and label reading, reinforcing rigidity, control, and obsessiveness leading to increased problems with eating.
Therapist suggestion:	"I was told by my other therapist to run up a hill as fast as I could to help with my anxiety after feeling fat when I ate."
Why it is not helpful:	While physical activity such as running and cardiovascular movement can be helpful for anxiety, people who have diagnosed eating disorders may have compromised physical health, especially if they have been severely restricting or throwing up food; the imbalance of electrolytes in their bodies in addition to strenuous exercise can increase their chance of severe issues with their heart that can be fatal. In addition, for many compulsive people over exercising is a problem and this suggestion feeds into unhealthy maintenance of their beliefs and reinforces these harmful behaviors.

Table 1.1 Signs of Possible Eating Disorder

Behavioral	Cognitive	Emotional	Psychological
• Fear around eating in the presence of others. • Feelings of undeserving, unworthy or needing to work for food. • Normal life is affected by food thoughts. • Avoiding events or situations where they may not be able to control food. • The need to plan meals before going out. • Inability for flexibility when eating out and needing to eat at specific restaurants or order specific food. • Constant comparison of own food to others food. • Constant comparison of body with others. • Feelings that others are judging what and how much they are eating. • Hypervigilance about what and how much others are eating • Constant body obsession and has an imagined ideal body image or weight for self. • Uses food rules and or restrictions. • Avoidance of people fearing judgment of their body. • Avoidance of activities that involve food and or exposure of body image. • Constant negative self • talk regarding body image. • Challenged when there are disruptions in their routine (the need to complete specific rituals, such as exercise routine, eating specific foods at certain times of the day) and causes distress. • Needing to compensate for food. It feels easier to eat only when they have exercised otherwise feels guilty for eating. • Experiences feelings such as guilt, shame, anger and or sadness after eating • Constant dieting or exploring latest food trends (fasting, trendy diets, miracle herbs and teas for weight management etc.) • Needing specific food (all organic, whole or raw foods etc.) and when not available causes distress or unable to eat anything else to fullness. • All other activities are scheduled around their exercise and food schedule.	• All or Nothing (black and white thinking) • Rumination • Negative self• talk • Obsessive/compulsive thoughts • Rigidity, inflexibility • Perfectionistic tendencies • Poor or foggy memory • Harsh and mean critical voice • ED voice (eating disorder voice) thoughts that encourage disordered eating behaviors • Overwhelming and cluttered thoughts • Constant doubting of self • Fearful and catastrophizing thoughts	• Has difficulty identifying their emotions • Difficulty with expressing emotions • Difficulty with tolerating uncomfortable feelings • Experiences anxiety or depression • Difficulty with being and needs to be kept busy or distracted • Struggles with staying present	• Sensitivity to rejection • Feelings of unworthiness ("I'm not enough") • Feeling undeserving • Tendency to compromise own beliefs for others in order to be accepted • Tends to avoid conflict or confrontation • Challenges around assertiveness communication and boundary setting • Challenges around communicating their own needs • High expectations from self • Fears judgment from others, constant self • judgment or judgment of others • Constant comparisons of self to others • Need to be liked by others • Hyper awareness of self or self • consciousness

Therapist suggestion: "I had come to some revelations with my individual therapist about how my eating disorder wasn't about food. I realized the function of my eating disorder. I shared my revelations with my group therapist at a program I was attending at the time, and the group therapist told me I was wrong, and that my eating disorder was all about the food."

Why it is not helpful: Clients in therapy discover and work on underlying issues that fuel their eating difficulties, learning how their eating problems have been functional in their lives. They discover that they've focused on distracting themselves by food, weight, and body image as a way of coping with uncomfortable feelings. When your client recognizes that it's not about the food, it shows your client making therapeutic progress and is willing to work through the real underlying problems.

Therapist suggestion: "My therapist told me it's normal to diet and want to lose weight. She said that she also goes on diets and wants to lose a few pounds, so she gave me the greenlight to continue."

Why it is not helpful: Normalizing behaviors for some clients can be helpful for specific issues. However, with eating disorders, individuals usually have a tendency to minimize problematic behaviors, and normalizing behaviors such as dieting or hyper fixating on weight loss gives the permission that your client is seeking to continue maladaptive behaviors. Some clients have an idea that their behaviors are maladaptive and are seeking a professional to confirm it. Therefore, if their behaviors are normalized, these clients view themselves as not "sick enough" and the obsessions will be more pronounced.

Therapist suggestion: "I was asked for weight loss tips by my therapist. She wanted my food and exercise routine, saying I was disciplined by the way I ate and it showed in my physical appearance."

Why it is not helpful: This may appear as a harmless compliment. However, commenting on their food behaviors and physical body activates their eating disorder voice, worsening and reinforcing their eating disorder. People may inadvertently make these comments towards your client not meaning harm. Therefore, your client will have to learn techniques to quiet these thoughts. However, when their therapist makes these comments, it can be detrimental to the therapeutic relationship and towards their entire treatment process.

Therapist suggestion: "My therapist told me to read all the labels and buy the foods I felt comfortable with. Of course, I didn't buy anything."

Why it is not helpful: Your client has a tendency to hyper fixate on numbers such as calories, weight, sizes, and food labels. Therefore, paying more attention to quantitative data allows for them to be more controlling around food and weight. The intention behind the suggestion may be to help your client feel comfortable with different foods, however, this usually exacerbates restrictive eating behaviors. It typically results in your client only purchasing their identified "safe foods." When they look at labels, clients will fixate on calories, ingredients, percentage of carbohydrates and fats. This gives them a sense of control and the rigidity of their thoughts will prevent food choice flexibility.

Most professionals who give the above suggestions do not understand eating disorders. They have not implemented an effective plan for their client to achieve recovery and this is where clients feel most frustrated with treatment which can cause ambivalence about recovery, therefore keeping them in their disorder.

No Approach Works for Everyone

Maladaptive eating behaviors and processes are unique to each person struggling with eating difficulties. Treatment is not a "one size fits all" approach but rather a "meet your client where they are at" approach. Individuals can have the same diagnosis, but the similarities stop there (Lazarus 1991). Therefore, every client must be treated individually, and clinicians need to be aware that some treatments come with limitations.

Of all mental health issues, eating disorders have arguably the highest number of contributing factors.

Here is a partial list of the many vulnerability and risk factors for eating disorders:

- Genetic and environmental factors.
- Cognitive distortions/ inflexibility, negative self-perception.

- Poor coping skills.
- Lack of human connection and support.
- Low self-esteem, low self-worth.
- Hypersensitivity.
- Interpersonal challenges.
- Lack of emotional distress tolerance.
- Perfectionism, obsessions.
- Alexithymia: difficulty recognizing emotions.
- Challenges with interoceptive awareness.
- Dieting, family eating habits, overeating.
- Trauma, depression, anxiety.
- Family dysfunction, problematic parenting and parental pathology.
- Shape and weight-related concerns, thin ideal.
- Family history of eating disorders.
- Dietary restraint, dieting.

People who struggle with eating issues are not only dealing with feelings around food, food behaviors, and body dissatisfaction. They are also challenged by stressful life events, unresolved trauma, loss, significant changes, family dysfunction, their negative thoughts and perceptions about themselves, their emotions, and their ability to tolerate uncomfortable emotions. They are dealing with a poor self-image, and this is intertwined with biological factors such as depression and anxiety. They may have difficulty with interpersonal relationships and other unresolved issues that have not yet been uncovered. To cope, your client may have decided to start a diet, manipulating what, when, and how they eat; studies show that dieting is a major contributor to developing an eating disorder (Stice et al. 2017.).

Your client has their own genetic predispositions that need to be considered which are influenced by their environment and life experiences. Therefore, if a contributing factor is missed in treatment, clients can easily relapse or the treatment will not be effective.

Eating disorders can transform and manifest in various ways.
Eating disorders can be everchanging, unpredictable, and vacillating. Eating disorders can also progressively worsen or transform into another type of eating disorder. For example, someone struggling with binge eating can develop bulimia nervosa, or an individual struggling with bulimia nervosa can transform into anorexia nervosa if all the root causes are not addressed and targeted. The treatment process is not linear.

A client's health can worsen without the appropriate level of care.
Determining the appropriate level of care can be tricky given what we have discussed about the complex nature of eating disorders. It manifests differently in each person and is dependent on the vulnerabilities, experiences, and background of each individual.

To make matters trickier, for example, clients may appear stable but may continue to restrict food whenever unsupervised. Or they may continue to avoid "fear foods" greatly impacting their life by prioritizing their day around the ability to make "safe food" choices. Careful assessment is vital in situations like these; these clients may need a level of care that can provide some practice around eating meals independently such as a partial hospitalization day program.

Some Clinicians Don't Realize that there is a Function for the Eating Disorder

At some point, you may have wondered, "why would anyone engage in behaviors that have no benefit for them?" Or more specifically, "why would my client binge and purge if all it does is harm them?" The truth is, all behaviors have a function. Even—or I like to say, *especially*—eating disorder behaviors.

Individuals use eating behaviors as a way of coping with or dealing with their present reality. There are many functions for an eating disorder, such as comfort, control, and relaxation just to give a few examples. It can be tricky to identify the function at first, which is another reason that eating disorders are complicated to treat. But over time a skilled therapist can pinpoint the function by decoding messages in their statements. Here are some examples of what clients have said to me and what the function might be for each.

"Food is my best friend." (Comfort)
"Restricting food makes me feel in control and strong." (Control)
"Purging food helps me feel cleaner and lighter." (Control)
"Bingeing on food helps me to fall asleep." (Relaxation or avoidance)

All behaviors have a function and when we can address the negative "unhelpful" function, the behavior can then be replaced with a positive "helpful" behavior that serves that particular function, or we could address the underlying cause of needing the function in the first place. Working through the underlying issue would then resolve the need to keep the issue hidden. Most eating issues mask the issue and keep it hidden.

Let's take a look at a basic process of what happens when someone is negatively emotionally activated and uses binge eating or restricting food as their maladaptive coping mechanism.

The different functions of disordered eating are unique to each individual. Eating disorders are developed in order to cope with areas in life that are highly stressful or to avoid situations all together. There are many ways that disordered eating can be used as maladaptive coping. For example, binging behaviors have a numbing effect and individuals engaging in this behavior typically disconnect from themselves, like flipping a switch and going onto auto pilot, feeling like the brain finally pauses until awareness of the present return, then guilt, shame, and disappointment set in.

Let's take a look at a case example that illustrates the functions that eating behaviors can serve.

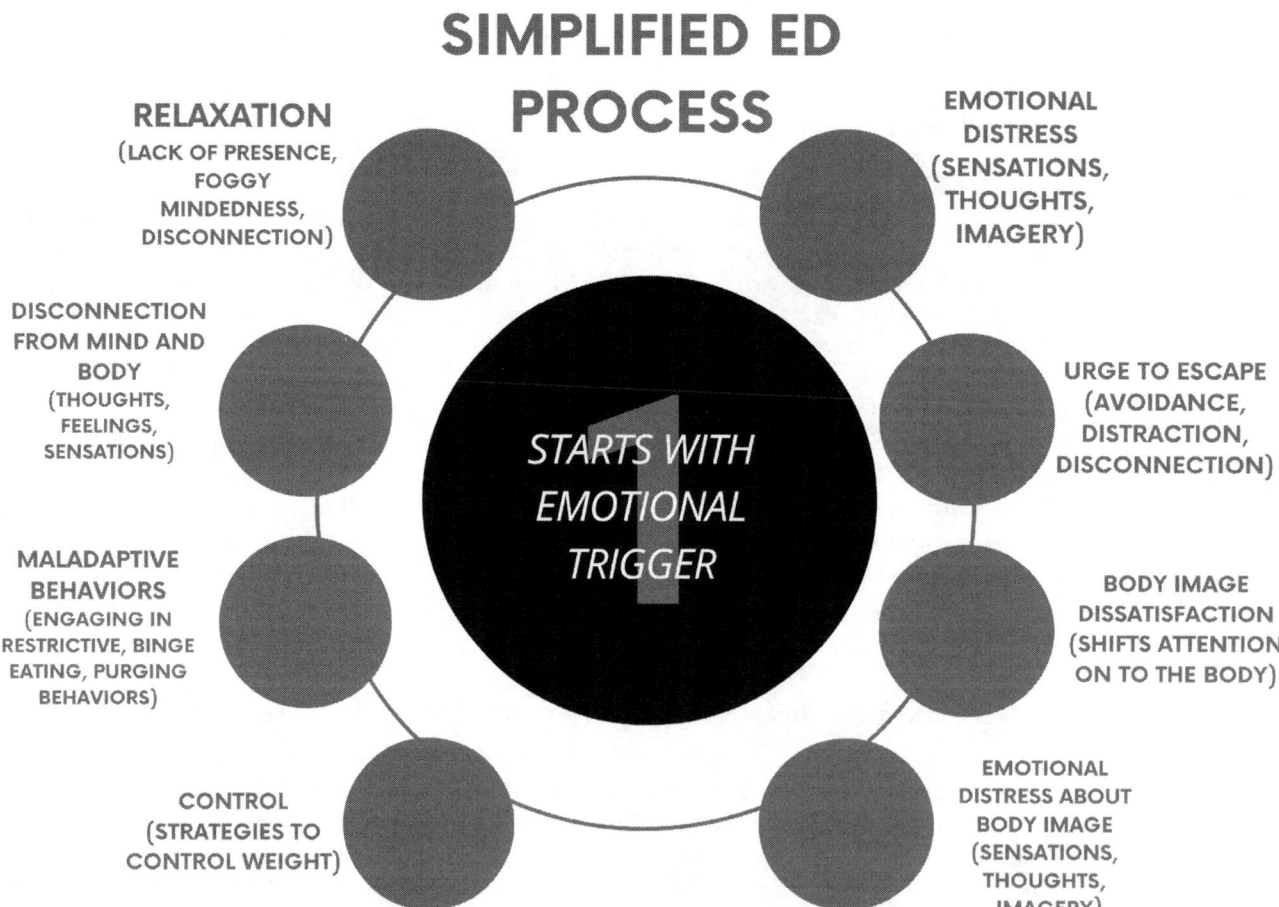

Figure 1.1 Simplified Disordered Eating Process

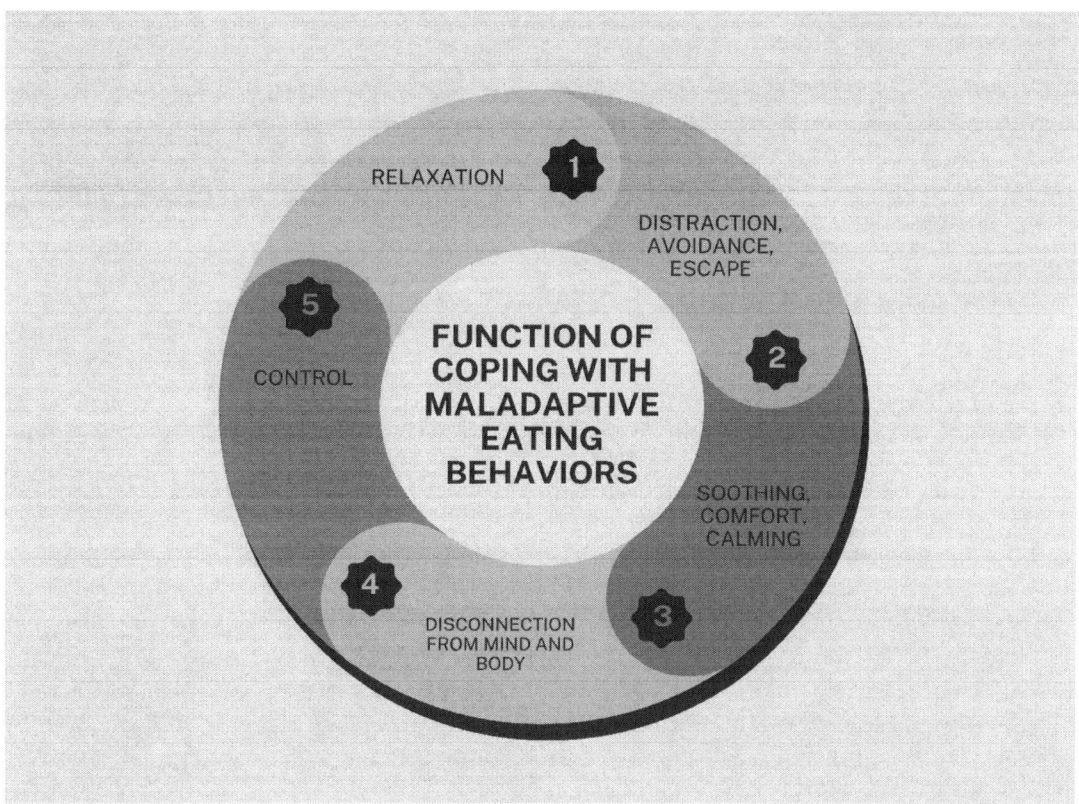

Figure 1.2 Function of Coping with Maladaptive Eating Behaviors

Function #1 Relaxation and Self Soothing

Kerri is a 39-year-old single professional woman seeking therapy for her issues regarding food, weight and body dissatisfaction. She's been working long hours and feels the need to work on holidays and weekends to relieve her co-workers. Kerri often feels resentment but *"it's the right thing to do."* Kerri is single and her co-workers have families. She often leaves work angry, and routinely relaxes and soothes herself with snacks in front of the television. *"I look forward to going home and just turning it all off."*

Function #2 Distraction

Kerri: *"Once I start, I can't stop. It's like my body is melted into the chair and I'm not paying any attention to what's on. My mind is blank and I'm in a zone. I don't even realize it's happening until the pain starts."*

When this process occurs, Kerri forgets about the anger and resentment from work. She is now completely distracted by the physical discomfort in her body.

Function #3 Control

Kerri: *"I have no willpower. I'm so angry at myself. I know better. But I guess I'll just get rid of it, or I won't eat as much for dinner, or I can skip breakfast and lunch."*

Kerri hasn't expressed her resentment about her situation at work and feels as though she doesn't have a choice or control over her work schedule. However, she has the ability to utilize behaviors as a way to cope even though the behaviors can be harmful to her. For example, eating both soothes her and becomes a distraction to the real issue (work schedule). Her anger about work is now covered with the anger towards herself for emotionally eating. This is not a conscious process. She may not have control over others at work, but she does have control over how she decides to cope.

Function # 4: Numbing

Kerri: *"I just shut everything out. I know I'm angry and hate that I feel upset. When I eat, it helps me to just numb out. I don't feel the anger anymore. Of course, I feel angry at myself for eating but that's my fault."*

Most People, Including Medical Professionals, Think Eating Disorders Are just about Food

Individuals that struggle with eating issues often hear from family and friends—and even well-meaning clinicians—statements such as:

> "Just stop eating when you're full."
> "Just eat."
> "Just don't buy the junk foods if you're going to eat it all."
> "Just lock the food up."
> "Just don't eat to the point where you think you'll purge it."
> "Just eat all good foods."
> "Just don't bring money with you."
> "Just eat in moderation."
> "Just diet and exercise."
> "Just drink lots of water."

What do all of these comments have in common? They help illustrate the point that the eating disorder is not just about food. Because if it were just about the food, individuals could follow a set of eating guidelines and there would be no other issues. In fact, individuals who struggle with eating issues are well versed in food and nutrition, reading labels, current diet trends, calories in food and diet supplements to name a few. They have researched food to the point that they could be experts in food nutrition themselves.

If the therapist believes the eating disorder is just about the food, it will be a frustrating process with the client believing it simply takes "will power" to make changes or to stop unwanted food behaviors. The client will likely question what is wrong with them and why they can't just do this. "If only I had enough will power/If only I were disciplined, then I wouldn't have this problem with food." These are common statements heard in therapy sessions when clients feel powerless and hopeless.

Therefore, therapists need to address the underlying issues and help the client understand what their food issues are about. Clients will lose their motivation for treatment if they feel the treatment is ineffective or unobtainable.

Eating disorders are not about the food initially but they become about the food.
When individuals struggle with eating food initially, it can be for many reasons such as:

- What the food represents for the individual.
- What the eating process represents for the individual.
- Eating behaviors are used as a coping mechanism by the individual.

However, when maladaptive behaviors such as restricting food, binging, and purging food result in medical complications that take a toll on the individual's mental and physical health, weight restoration and medical stability become the primary focus. This is normally addressed in a higher level of care treatment such as inpatient hospitalization, or residential care. Only after the individual is medically stable and functioning cognitively within normal limits can psychotherapy be effective. This is an example of when eating problems become about the food and when the client will need to adhere to treatment protocols regarding eating as prescribed by their medical team.

Most People, Including Medical Professionals, Mistakenly Believe that Body Dissatisfaction Is only about the Body

Cultural and social influences strongly affect our clients' body image ideals. These learned ideals become their personal goals. We are inundated by images across billboards, magazines, movies, television, and social media. The societal ideal about how the body should appear carries the message that our lives will magically improve if we look a certain way, because people who embody this standard—we are promised and come to believe—are happier, more powerful, more successful, and envied by all others. The goal then becomes to transform one's body to resemble whoever the media has named the "It" person of the moment. With these ubiquitous messages about body, it's easy to see how a young person would naturally attach their worth or value to their looks—and come up with the belief that changing their body could be a solution to their problem of not feeling good about themselves or needing to feel accepted. Their perceived flaws—whether it's the shape of their body, their weight, or something else—are then used as tangible evidence about what they feel is wrong with them.

Regrettably, therapists may neglect to address the deeper issues when their client is feeling dissatisfied with their body: Most treatments are about teaching individuals about body acceptance. Teaching body acceptance is paramount for eating disorder recovery however, it is only part of the solution in dealing with body image struggles. Trends about physical attractiveness will continue to exist and influence our clients. It is a billion-dollar industry that makes financial gains from people dissatisfied with their bodies. The "promise" of whatever they are marketing is what individuals will continue to seek. Therefore, it is not about the physical body and trends. It is about the "promise", the declaration or assurance that a particular thing will happen that the client is after. Therapists will need to address the "promise." This is part of the underlying issue that the client will need to work through.

If it were only about their physical body, then theoretically once individuals reach their perceived ideal weight, they would feel better about themselves and who they are, right? Well, anyone who works with eating disorders knows that this isn't true. Once individuals get to that weight, they are usually dissatisfied and have a new goal weight or physical appearance goal. This will be addressed more in depth in Chapter 7, *Exploring Body Neutrality and Acceptance.*

Case example: Kerri: Body dissatisfaction and what it represents

Kerri: *"I've never been in a long-term relationship. Sometimes, I wonder what's wrong with me? I don't think anyone will want to be with me."*

Therapist: *"What makes you think that no one will want to be with you?"*

Kerri: *"Well, I'm a middle-aged single woman. Isn't that enough evidence. I'm not exactly in high demand."*

At 39, most of Kerri's friends are married and have families. She spends most of her time at work and her co-workers are also married. For the first time Kerri fears being alone and never finding a life partner. Lately, her body image dissatisfaction has increased and she fears not being physically attractive. *"Men don't want a 39-year-old woman. They want some woman in her 20s. I hate that I've aged and the way my skin looks."* Therefore, her physical body represents the potential of being alone for the rest of her life. She squeezes the skin from her belly and says, *"this is evidence that I'm not attractive and that no one will want me."*

Kerri has issues with her physical body because of what her physical body represents. She fears being alone for the rest of her life and her perception of her physical body is the evidence that no one will want to be with her. Therefore, her physical body represents the obstacle that keeps others from wanting a meaningful long-term relationship with her.

Failure to Address the Eating Disorder Voice Can Sabotage the Recovery Process

Eating disorder thoughts and voice can be tricky to recognize because the eating disorder voice can be convincingly persuasive especially when it appears that your client is doing well. Often it is difficult for therapists to recognize that some of our clients' desires may be inspired by values that align with and preserve their eating disorder. Your client may even be unaware that their desire may be driven from a place that helps sustain their eating disorder. Therefore, it is our job as their therapist to be able to recognize these tricky thoughts, requests, or behaviors quickly so that they can be addressed. These behaviors can help maintain your client's eating disorder and sabotage their recovery if not acknowledged. Your client may not be aware of this and genuinely feel that their requests are in support of their recovery. However, when your client is further into their recovery process and using their skills, they will be able to recognize how these requests are part of refusing to let go of all behaviors in order to continue to use some parts of disordered eating to feel safe. Below are some examples of how these tricky behaviors show up and how it interferes with your client's recovery process.

1. *Measuring food*: It is common for clients that struggle with food restriction to want to keep measuring their food. They often give reasons such as "I want to make sure I'm getting enough." While this sounds like it makes sense and that your client is recovery minded, most often it isn't the case. Measuring food allows the client to feel in control of their food and portions sizes, making sure that they are not inadvertently giving themselves more than they have to. This is still a form of control and doesn't allow for the client to work through feelings related to ambiguity from not measuring food. They are not able to let go of obsessions around food, calories, and portion sizes. Clients that have a tendency to restrict their calories know exactly how many calories are in certain portions and measuring food will keep them from full recovery from their eating disorder if not addressed.

2. *Reading Labels*: Similar to measuring food, some clients will have a tendency to continue to read food labels, "I want to make sure it doesn't have any ingredients that make me sick." Some will claim that they have food sensitivities so that they can continue to read labels. This helps them stay in control, know portion sizes, calories, and fat and carb grams and again will keep them from completely recovering from their eating disorder.

3. *I felt sick so I made myself throw up*: Some individuals will tell you that they didn't purge, but induced vomiting so that they could feel better physically. "*I felt the food heavy in my chest, and it felt like a brick. I wasn't purging. I just felt sick and knew I'd feel better, if I got rid of it.*" This appears as though the client knows the difference between a purge and can differentiate when they're feeling physically sick, however, most people don't induce vomiting when they are genuinely sick. When people experience nausea, the vomiting is an involuntary process. This is a way to continue to engage in purging and to keep a part of the eating disorder. The therapist will need to address the underlying issues that is causing the client to purge.

Clients Often Misreport Their Well-Being, Leading to an Ineffective Treatment Plan

Your client may appear happy and healthy, their weight may appear normal, and they may report that they are okay. However, if you dive deeper, you may discover that they are engaging in restrictive behaviors, or obsessed with food. They may be focused on their body and or maybe, dieting, intermittent fasting, or taking diet pills, laxatives or diuretics. They may not only be restricting food but also things like money and relationships. Clients can also be struggling with binging on food but can also binge on relationships, work, alcohol, shopping etc.

Clients may insist they're on a "healthy" diet. Some clients may tell you that they have decided to be vegetarian or start veganism for the love of animals, or to protect the earth. While they may naturally have these values, if these changes were made at the start of their eating disorder, this can be part of their problematic eating process, and over time, they will continue to cut out other foods and maintain restrictive eating. Many, as they get stronger in their recovery, will acknowledge that they cut out certain foods due to the eating disorder rather than out of the beliefs they stated earlier. They will then add variety back into their normal diet.

Clients with eating disorders often know more about food and nutrition than the average psychotherapist. For this reason, it's common for clients to use research articles as evidence to strengthen the eating disorder. Clients will often use the argument, "See, how am I supposed to get better when even the research shows that thinner more attractive people have better opportunities." Other examples include, "processed foods are bad for you, so I should only eat healthy foods" or "There many health benefits for fasting and its coming from medical professionals, so there's nothing wrong with me fasting." These topics needs to be addressed as people who struggle with eating disorders can often get fixated on these ideas and it is used to fuel the eating disorder and maintains maladaptive behaviors.

Clients may insist they have allergies or food sensitivities. It is common for people who struggle with eating issues to hyper fixate on what they feel in their bodies. For many, they're sensitive to uncomfortable sensations or changes in their bodies after eating. They may experience bloating, indigestion, or other symptoms that they may seek out help for. They may learn that they have food sensitivities, and this can encourage disordered eating thoughts to worsen, because it can cause clients to be hypervigilant about what they're eating, worsening problematic eating behaviors.

For example, generally, someone has a food sensitivity without disordered eating may decide to avoid from bread or pasta because of how it affects them. They may experience digestive issues, inflammation, or medical issues. However, they may eat rice or potatoes. In contrast, someone with an eating disorder may believe they have a food sensitivity, may read all labels and hyper fixate on what they are eating. Eating becomes something they fear, and they may choose to cut out categories such as all starchy carbohydrates.

Clients may insist on a return to "normal" life activities. When clients have been in recovery from their eating disorder it's common for them to want to return to "normal" activities and engage in their life again as it was, for example, intuitive eating, fasting for religious reasons, modeling, or a competitive sport. Eventually returning to normal is what recovery is all about. However, when someone has a history of eating disorder and has for example struggled with compulsive over exercise or a tendency to obsess over losing weight, we have to be cautious about their motivations behind the desire to do things that can potentially sabotage their recovery. For example, your client may express the desire to return to the gym, run a marathon, compete in a body building competition, return to ballet or competitive dancing. While this may sound benign, this can be the start of the unraveling of their eating disorder recovery.

The client may appear that they are in a good place in their recovery but without a solid foundation for their recovery your client will likely relapse. This is due to what "competitive" means. When someone is competing they're in it to win it, therefore mindfulness, listening to what their body needs, honoring rest, and all the important concepts needed for eating disorder recovery are ignored. Another common example (usually from clients who have a tendency to restrict food) is that they would like to "not think about food anymore." They may say something like, "Normal people don't have to think about food all the time. I don't want to have to think about food. I just want to eat when I'm hungry, instead of having to think about my meals." This may be their way of avoiding accountability with meals and having to eat regularly when they haven't quite mastered intuitive eating, and this can be a red flag for a backslide in their recovery.

While the goal is eventually returning to a form of normalcy, and to be able to intuitively listen to their body and eat when their body is hungry, most that have restricted eating for many years will have challenges with their body cues. Therefore, it is important that they are following structured eating (as directed by their nutritionist or dietitian) until they are ready to fully practice intuitive eating.

What Treatment Approach Is Best?

Eating disorders are complex and need to be treated in a way that will target all of the problematic areas. As each client is unique, the approach needs to be customized to meet their needs.

On average, approximately, 70% of people struggling with eating disorders will relapse at least once (Miskovic-Wheatley et al. 2023.) because they have failed to learn adaptive ways to cope with life's stressors. They seek out immediate gratification to resolve uncomfortable emotions or physical bodily sensations. This is the cause of relapse. As a result, many use their eating disorder as a placeholder as a way to cope until real underlying issues are uncovered and identified and dealt with. Using substances or maladaptive behaviors to numb, avoid, or distract are normalized. These coping styles are often glamorized in movies, social media, and through social circles. Seeking help for emotional distress is often viewed as a weakness which prevents individuals from talking or sharing their pain with others, instead seeking out other maladaptive ways to cope with their suffering.

Unfortunately, most therapists (who may lack training because none was offered) still operate under these misconceptions. I'll say it again: One of the most insidious misconceptions about eating disorders is that they're only about food. Sadly, this leads to a very narrow treatment approach that rarely yields long-term recovery. To illustrate this, let's look at a treatment plan written by a well-intentioned therapist who asked me to review it for her client diagnosed with bulimia nervosa. The client was instructed to follow this plan when she had urges to engage in her binge and purge cycle.

1. Eat normally.
2. Accept your body. Be positive.
3. Use a coping skill.
4. Do self-care.
5. Be kind to yourself.

This doesn't look too off the mark, right? Unfortunately, her client was not making progress, therefore, she was referred to me. I asked Rebecca, 19, how the plan was working out for her. Here's what she shared with me.

"When I get into the mindset that I'm going to eat there's no stopping me. I may look at the plan, but it means nothing to me. I don't know what 'eat normally' looks like. I always start out with a careful portion, but then I get to this point where it's like something takes over and I can't stop until the food is all gone. I go through the pantry and I feel almost like I'm in a trance. I can't stop."

"I want to accept my body but to be honest, I feel so gross after I eat. I'm bloated and feel so sick, like I'm going to explode. There's just no way I'm going to be positive. I hate myself. I feel so ashamed and guilty. I hate it and just don't know what's wrong with me."

"When I'm in the zone of eating, I can't stop and think that I'm going to use a coping tool. That's the furthest thing from my mind. It feels intense and nothing is going to make me stop in that moment."

The plan is not wrong but it lacks the specific skills needed to achieve these goals. For the therapist, these goals may seem easily achievable. However, Rebecca has no idea how to go about doing any of these things, especially if she has been engaging in problematic eating behaviors for a while. Rebecca doesn't know what "eat normally" means. How would Rebecca go about just eating normally or just accepting her body?

It's common for people with eating problems to struggle to identify coping skills that work for them. Due to the nature of this disorder (the function of the disorder is to decrease consciousness) many have not found other coping skills that are more effective than their eating disorder. Eating behaviors are used to cope with underlying issues beneath the surface that the client has been avoiding and will require help from a therapist to identify more effective coping tools.

Rebecca is seeking immediate relief from whatever uncomfortable emotions or sensations she is dealing with, and binging and purging has been the most effective for her. It would be almost impossible for Rebecca to just give up her most effective tool and choose something different without specific skills and guidance from her therapist.

Yes, it is important to address Rebecca's body dissatisfaction and it's also important to address food behaviors. However, when therapists do this without addressing the reasons for the client's dissatisfaction or why they are using the food behaviors, it prevents both the therapist and client from uncovering the real reasons behind the client's dissatisfaction, leaving both to feel stuck.

Therapists have to address behaviors around eating and also the underlying issues. This should be an integrated approach that addresses the whole body. For example, individuals need to learn how to connect to their bodies and how to differentiate physical hunger from emotional hunger. Individuals also need to learn how their thoughts affect their behaviors, the origins of their thoughts, and their judgment and how it affects their self-perception and contributes to their emotional distress.

The challenges that therapists face in working with people who struggle with eating problems are the very aspects that our clients utilize in order to maintain their eating disorder. Therefore, what this tells us is that our clients fear losing the only effective coping mechanism they know for dealing with life's hardships. The basic assumptions we can make from this are as follows.

Individuals struggling with eating issues haven't been able to find adaptive ways to cope with their challenges. Therefore, our clients need be taught specific foundational skills to deal with life and its hardships and learn new responses so that they are able to adapt with the life's unexpected difficulties, ultimately replacing eating behaviors as a way of coping, and making it possible for the therapist to address the real underlying issues.

What if I told you that your client's eating process, behaviors, food choices, how and what they eat are all essential information for a lasting recovery? What if I told you that helping someone recover from an eating disorder can be less complicated than you think? What if I told you that you could learn to understand what your client needs or feels by asking about what they ate and the process by which they ate the food in that week? These are all part of the nine foundational skills that I will introduce to you in Chapter 2. Your client will need to learn these essential skills as part of the Integrative Approach. This multimodal framework addresses your client as a unique individual and identifies your clients' needs for lasting eating disorder recovery.

Bibliography

Lazarus, C. N. (1991). Conventional diagnostic nomenclature versus multimodal assessment. *Psychological Reports, 68,* 1363–1367.

Miskovic-Wheatley, J., Bryant, E., Ong, S. H. *et al.* (2023). Eating disorder outcomes: findings from a rapid review of over a decade of research. *Journal of Eating Disorders, 11,* 85. https://doi.org/10.1186/s40337-023-00801-3.

Sala, M., Keshishian, A., Song, S., Moskowitz, R., Bulik, C. M., Roos, C. R., & Levinson, C. A. (2023). Predictors of relapse in eating disorders: A meta-analysis. *Journal of Psychiatric Research, 158,* 281–299. https://doi.org/10.1016/j.jpsychires.2023.01.002.

Silén, Y., & Keski-Rahkonen, A. (2022). Worldwide prevalence of DSM-5 eating disorders among young people. *Current Opinion in Psychiatry, 35*(6), 362–371. https://doi.org/10.1097/YCO.0000000000000818.

Stice, E., Gau, J. M., Rohde, P., & Shaw, H. (2017). Risk factors that predict future onset of each DSM-5 eating disorder: Predictive specificity in high-risk adolescent females. *Journal of Abnormal Psychology, 126*(1), 38–51. https://doi.org/10.1037/abn0000219.

Striegel Weissman, R., & Rosselli, F. (2017). Reducing the burden of suffering from eating disorders: Unmet treatment needs, cost of illness, and the quest for cost-effectiveness. *Behaviour Research and Therapy, 88,* 49–64. https://doi.org/10.1016/j.brat.2016.09.006.

Chapter 2

Treating the Person

How do you begin to help your client with their eating problems? Where do you start if there are multiple challenges? Should you start with regulating food or with regulating emotions? Say you decide to help with regulating food, how do you go about it? Your client is feeling hopeless and out of control with their eating behaviors. They are feeling discouraged and don't know how to stop. What would your strategy be to help them stop the cycle? If your client is engaging in a vicious cycle of eating behaviors, more than likely they are also going through emotional suffering, defeatism, and experiencing a pessimistic outlook about their life.

When a client calls for an appointment or comes in for their first session, our first priority is to ensure that the client is getting the right kind of help. This means that it is important that the appropriate level of care is identified. More often than not, your client will likely be struggling in ways that aren't life-threatening but are serious nevertheless. Remember, eating disorders affect all domains of a person's being, biologically, psychologically, emotionally, socially, spiritually, and interpersonally and it is important to help your clients choose other ways to cope .

Multimodal Treatment Approach

Arnold Lazarus developed the multimodal treatment approach as a comprehensive biopsychosocial framework in dealing with the complexities and uniqueness of people. This model is key because it takes in account of the multitude of factors affecting the individual. Using this framework means important aspects of how eating disorders develop, their prevention, treatment, and recovery are not missed.

The *biological* elements include genetics, bone structure, body composition, and genetic predisposition to depression and anxiety including OCD and any issues that are biological in nature. The *psychological* aspects include (social and emotional and behavioral components) self-esteem, feelings of self-worth, perfectionism, control, poor sense of self, and inability to create boundaries and assertively communicate. Finally, the *social* components include social status, socioeconomics, family and cultural influences such as cultural expectations, and social media. We know how biological factors can influence our genetics and our predisposition for certain vulnerabilities, but our environment in our upbringing, family, peers, community, culture, society, and the world also play a major role in how we are and how we perceive ourselves.

This approach addresses the whole person often missed in single therapeutic approaches. Arnold Lazarus's comprehensive framework utilizes a comprehensive biopsychosocial assessment—in this book referred to as the Multimodal Treatment Assessment (MMT), which I adapted for eating disorders. Hence, in addition to focusing on behavior, cognition, and affect, MMT also thoroughly assesses imagery, sensations, interpersonal relationships, and biological factors, resulting in a seven-point assessment framework called the BASIC I.D.

Given that the most common biological intervention is the use of psychotropic drugs, the first letters from the seven modalities can be combined to produce the convenient acronym "BASIC I.D." although the "D" modality actually represents the complete range of physiological and biological factors beyond the use of substances, prescribed or otherwise. Hence, the BASIC I.D. refers to:

- Behavior (our actions).
- Affect (our emotions).
- Sensation (our senses).

DOI: 10.4324/9781032651408-4

- Imagery (our ability to visualize, imagine, and think in pictures).
- Cognition (our language-based thinking).
- Interpersonal relationships (our intimate connections and other social involvements).
- Drugs (our physical bodies, health behaviors, and medical matters).

BASIC I.D. not only provides for comprehensive and highly individualistic problem identification, but also connotes peoples' uniqueness—their "basic identity" (Lazarus 2019) making this a truly integrated approach that treats the whole person.

I've adapted Lazarus's integrative, multimodal model for assessing eating disorders. Here's what it looks like, with a few examples from Nicole, from Chapter 1.

B: Behavioral

Food behaviors such as restricting, binging, and purging food (plus overcompensating behaviors such as self-induced vomiting, excessive exercising, laxative, and diuretic use) help individuals to distract from or numb and ultimately avoid their painful reality. Their pain commonly consists of underlying fears such as conflict, rejection, failure, responsibility, or loneliness. Clients normally have limited insight as to why they are using these behaviors; they can only articulate the surface reasons, such as weight loss, in order to feel better about themselves. For example, Nicole shared, "*I didn't eat because I don't feel deserving of food. I feel like such a failure and maybe if I can lose weight, I'll feel better about myself.*"

A: Affect/Emotional

Individuals who struggle with eating issues have a lower emotional distress tolerance and baseline; and they commonly struggle with *alexithymia*, a condition that makes it more challenging for individuals to recognize what they are experiencing emotionally. Nicole had been using purging as a coping tool to deal with her emotional distress, anxiety, and anger. She struggled to recognize and acknowledge her feelings because expressing feelings wasn't acceptable in her family. Growing up, no one in her family could teach her how to deal with feelings. Nicole had an emotionally absent father that used alcohol to cope and her mother enabled her father's maladaptive behaviors.

S: Sensing/Physical Sensations

People who struggle with eating issues have difficulty with noticing and connecting to subtle physical sensations so unless these sensations are intense and obvious, they are likely ignored. This is the reason people who struggle with eating have trouble recognizing their physical hunger and fullness cues. Often these sensations have been ignored due to other intolerable associations, such as trauma held in their body or painful memories. Our clients disengage from their bodies so that they avoid these unbearable experiences. Often our clients have difficulty with interoceptive awareness, being able to sense and perceive the internal state of their bodies. For example, it's quite common for our clients to ignore their body's need for rest or physical activity. This is exacerbated by your client's tendency to tune into harsh, critical, and obsessive thoughts instead.

I: Imagery

When your client struggles with negative cognitions, it often triggers emotions and distress, which can then activate your client to imagine worst-case scenarios. This results in increased negative thoughts and intolerable emotional distress. Your client may also be dealing with flashbacks or troubling memories triggered by any of the other modalities. Imagery is an important domain that can affect your client's urges to use maladaptive coping and can affect the recovery progress if not addressed. For example, Nicole spoke about imagining her boyfriend dating someone else, and this vision was causing her urges to throw up. The images triggered her negative self-talk, causing her to create and hold on to unhelpful stories that kept her from moving forward, leading to extreme emotional distress.

This domain also includes aspects of your client's sense of purpose, beliefs, and spirituality that keep them stuck or feeling hopeless about their future or their recovery. People who struggle with eating issues often feel lost because they also struggle with knowing what they want and need. As mentioned earlier, pleasing others to avoid conflict is commonplace. Helping our clients connect to something bigger than themselves allows healing, rediscovery of self, and how to make self-centering changes to live a more purposeful life.

C: Cognitive

When clients are severely restricting calories or avoiding specific foods, such as carbohydrates, a lack of nutrition may affect their memory, focus, and ability to track cognitively. This is also true for clients who are purging. People who struggle with eating also exhibit rigidity in their thinking and frequently experience negative thinking. These negative cognitions contribute to a loud critical inner voice, self-deprecating thoughts, and punitive self-talk.

These negative thinking patterns occupy ample and boundless space in your client's mind, resulting in poor concentration, lack of presence, and emotional exhaustion. Eventually they can become paralyzing and debilitating, causing your client to lose motivation and hope that their situation can improve. This can be a trigger for them to utilize food behaviors in order to quiet the negative thoughts or to distract from the relentlessness of harsh critical thoughts. However, soon the negative thoughts resurface because of the emotional distress and feeling of shame and guilt that comes with using food behaviors—and this triggers the cycle to start again.

I: Interpersonal

Humans are wired for close connections, sense of belonging, safety, and attunement. Therefore, the inability to create long-lasting gratifying relationships is directly related to the experiences of early attachment. Individuals who struggle with eating issues have a higher probability of disruption in their attachment with primary caregivers than others so your client may have problematic and complex family dynamics. They may not have learned interpersonal skills, and may tend to choose to isolate. This is problematic, because connection with others is key to recovering from an eating disorder. Clients will need to understand their attachment style in order to heal old childhood wounds. This also helps them to understand how their lack of attachment, safety, and attunement can hamper their own ability to self-soothe and self-regulate.

D: Biological/Neurological

People who are vulnerable to using eating as a way of coping commonly have a genetic predisposition to depression or anxiety and may have family members who also struggle with this. It is also common for individuals who struggle with eating issues to have OCD or other disorders. This is important because a physician overseeing any medical or biological concerns, such as medication management or medical conditions, will be part of your client's multidisciplinary treatment team.

Four-Part Process for Sustained Recovery

Utilizing Lazarus' model, and as a result working with this population extensively for more than 20 years, I've developed an effective four-part process towards sustained eating disorder recovery using various dependable techniques to achieve the most effective results.

1. **Establishing a relationship and getting to know your client:** First, you'll need to conduct a comprehensive biopsychosocial assessment. Using the Multimodal Treatment Assessment, which has been adapted for eating disorders, below, you can examine the seven modalities in your client's process: behavior, affect, sensations, imagery, cognition, interpersonal, biological/neurological. This will help you to understand what your client uniquely needs.
2. **Creating awareness about underlying issues through decoding metaphors:** Then you will help your client build and cultivate a strong skills foundation using the exercises, worksheets, and tools found in the next chapters. You will teach your client the foundational skills in the order that benefits them the most based on their needs.
3. **Revealing the function of the ED and uncovering underlying issues below the surface:** Next, you'll help your client understand why they are engaging in disordered eating, thus revealing the function of the disordered behaviors, and at the same time helping your client gain awareness about the underlying issues.

4. **Using a multimodality treatment approach:** Finally (this is happening simultaneously through the four phases) you'll help your client to recognize, practice, and apply the foundational skills in their everyday life while working to resolve the real underlying issues, therefore, eliminating the basis of their eating disorder.

The third step reveals the function of the eating disorder and creates client consciousness. This is often a pivotal moment for clients and can be the turning point in their treatment. They tend to view their eating disorder a little differently and can start to have more compassion towards themselves because this multimodal treatment approach is essentially focused on what they need.

Part 1: Establishing a Relationship and Getting to Know Your Client

Conduct a Comprehensive Biopsychosocial Assessment

In this multimodal treatment approach, the comprehensive biopsychosocial assessment is a key component of the template used to address the unique needs of your client. This assessment is an essential piece to understanding your client and will be your guide in determining the order in which your client needs to learn essential skills.

Priority is given to the biological modality to rule out clinical depression or effects of debilitating anxiety. Your client may require medication for chemical imbalances and need to be treated by a physician as part of the multimodal approach.

CLINICIAN WORKSHEET: MULTIMODAL TREATMENT ASSESSMENT

This assessment targets the seven modalities of the BASIC I.D., developed by Arnold Lazarus. The questions have been modified to apply to eating disorders. These modalities are in no way linear or static but exist in reciprocal transaction.

B: Behavioral

- What behaviors is your client engaging in related to food, weight, body image that is interfering with their life satisfaction (relationships, work, school?) (self-defeating actions, maladaptive behaviors)?
- What helpful behaviors does your client need to learn in order to increase adaptive or decrease maladaptive behaviors?
- What behaviors does your client need to start or stop doing?
- How do these behaviors affect the other modalities? (For example: obsessing over weight affects focus at work, and affects cognitive, imagery, and interpersonal domains.)
- How do these eating behaviors affect your client's daily functioning?

A: Affect

- What are your client's predominant emotions (affective reactions) around food, weight, and body image?
- What is your client dealing with in their emotions? Anger, anxiety, depression, sadness, envy, grief?
- What extent is your client experiencing (ex: irritation, versus rage; sadness versus profound melancholy)?
- What appears to generate these negative emotions, certain cognitions, images, interpersonal conflicts?
- How does your client respond (behave) when feeling a certain emotion?
- What impact do various behaviors have on your client?
- How do your client's emotions affect the other modalities?
- How do your client's emotions (affective reactions) affect their daily functioning?

S: Sensing

- Does your client experience specific sensory complaints (e.g., tension, chronic pain, tremors)?
- What physical sensations does your client experience in their body?
- What feelings, thoughts, and behaviors are connected to these bodily sensations?

- What positive or negative sensations (e.g., visual, auditory, tactile, olfactory, gustatory) does your client report?
- Does your client experience any physical sensations related to sensuality or sexuality or intimacy?
- Do any of the physical sensations affect other modalities?
- How do these physical sensations affect your client's daily functioning?

I: Imagery

- What fantasies and images are predominant for your client?
- What is your client's self-perception?
- What does your client visualize about themselves?
- What are your client's predominant images related to?
- What are your client's negative or intrusive images (e.g., flashbacks, unhappy or traumatic experiences)?
- How have these images or fantasies become obstacles preventing your client from creating newer, more helpful healing images?
- How are these images connected to ongoing cognitions, behaviors, and affective reactions?
- How do your client's images and fantasies affect other modalities and how do the images affect your client's daily functioning?
- What are your client's beliefs, values around spirituality?
- What are your client's goals, perceptions, desires, passions, and sense of purpose?

C: Cognitions

- What are your client's main attitudes, values, beliefs and opinions about food, weight, and body image?
- What are your client's predominant expectations of themselves such as "I should", or "I must?"
- What dysfunctional beliefs or irrational ideas does your client have related to food, weight, and body image?
- What negative automatic thoughts does your client experience?
- What are some of your client's negative thought patterns around food, weight, and body image?
- How do these patterns affect your client? How does your client perceive their cognitions?
- How does it affect other modalities and their daily functioning?

D: Biological/Neurological

- What medical and/or health issues does your client experience?
- Does your client have any medical concerns?
- What details pertain to nutrition, weight, sleep, exercise, alcohol, and drug use?
- How does your client view their health?
- How does your client feel their health is affecting other domains and in daily functioning?

Determine where to Start with Skills Foundation

In the following chapters, I've ordered the nine foundational skills by what I have found to be most beneficial to clients. However, based on using the Multimodal Treatment Assessment, you will determine the order in which you will teach them these skills. It is not the approach that drives their recovery but what your client needs for their recovery. The nine foundational skills were developed specifically for your client to equip them with the skills to cope through all areas listed in BASIC I.D.

Eventually your clients will be able to work through the underlying issues that fuel their eating disorder. The skills help them understand what is happening and why they are using their eating disorder as a way of coping. The skills also help increase your client's awareness and helps them to feel in control because they will have a plan and tools to use.

These foundational skills will become the anchor for your clients and act as a guide to help them stay mindful and conscious. Remember, the key to lasting eating disorder recovery is consciousness. With this, they will notice when they are approaching a slippery slope and use the skills needed to help them maintain their recovery and prevent relapse. Without this awareness, clients may miss the first hints of trouble, spiral, and potentially relapse, unless they are able to utilize the foundational skills.

The Nine Foundational Skills for Eating Disorder Recovery

I identified the nine foundational skills for eating disorder recovery through my own experience in working with clients who sustained long term eating disorder recovery. De Vos et al.'s research review showed the strongest indicators for eating disorder recovery (De Vos et al. 2017). Positive relationships with others, self-acceptance, autonomy, personal growth, improved eating disorder behavior and cognitions, and self-adaptability and resilience were the main components that recovered individuals shared. This confirmed what I had observed in the clients that I have treated.

Other criteria for sustained eating disorder recovery identified by the study included individuals having an improved body image evaluation, social contribution, purpose and meaning in life, spiritual integration, overall improved functioning, and positive affect.

Each of the nine essential skills are discussed chapter by chapter, including exercises and worksheets to develop these skills in your clients. However, as mentioned earlier, the Multimodal Treatment Assessment and your work with your client will dictate the order in which you would like to introduce each skill to them. These skills build on one another and are applied synchronously. Therefore, just as the modalities are reciprocal and transactional and don't follow a linear or static process, the foundational skills work in the same way. You will notice that the nine foundational skills incorporate and target various challenges found in the seven modalities with which your client may be struggling.

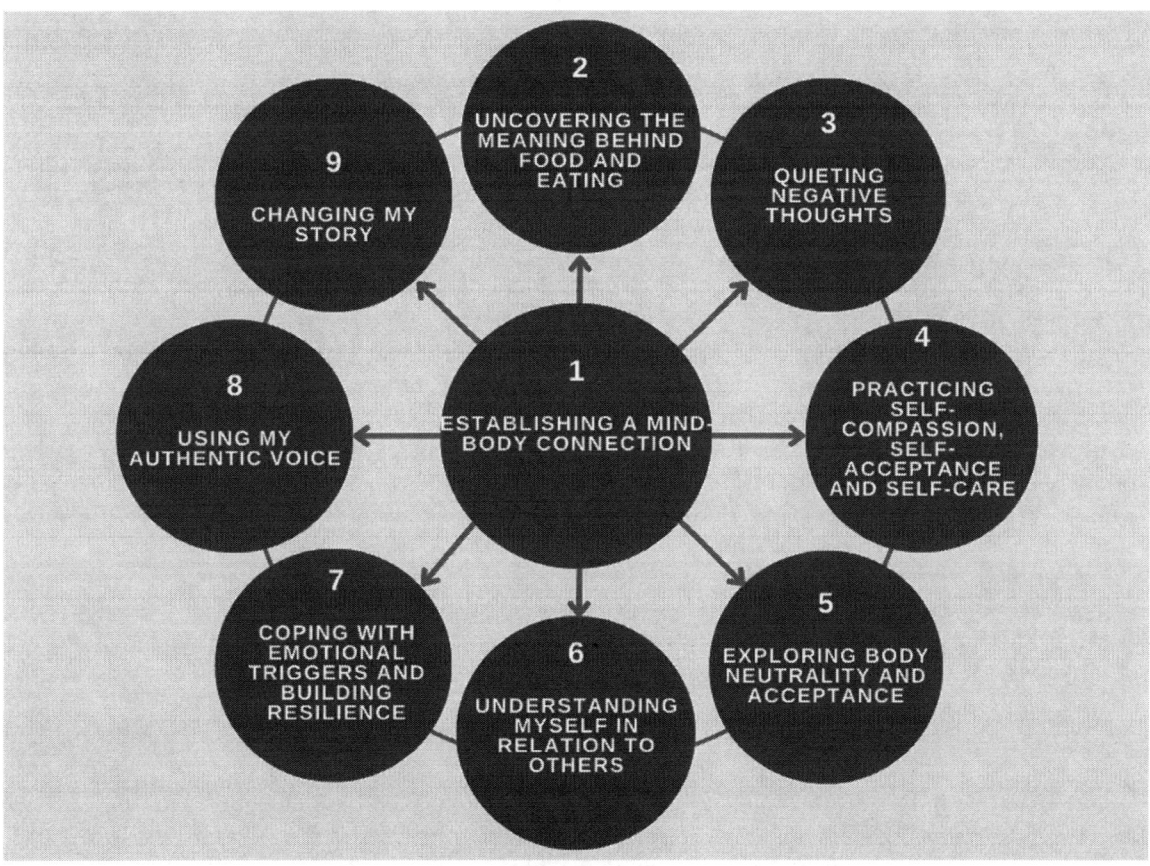

Figure 2.1 Nine Foundational Skills

1. **Establishing a mind-body connection (Chapter 3):** The first foundational skill incorporates several modalities from the multimodal therapy framework. This skill is extremely important because people who have eating disorders have learned to disconnect from their bodies in order to avoid experiencing uncomfortable emotions and physical sensations. Disconnecting from their bodies means they rarely notice cues, signals, intuition and messages—including hunger and fullness—unless they are blatantly obvious. Part of the reconnection process that your client will undergo is learning to listen to their bodies and honor what their bodies need. In order for your client to recover from their ED, this foundational skill is paramount.

2. **Uncovering the meaning behind food and eating (Chapter 4):** This skill helps your client learn what they truly need by learning to interpret the meaning behind their food behaviors and emotional hunger. Learning this foundational skill helps them recognize that their problem has little to do with food. Rather, the food or eating behaviors have come to symbolize the true issue that lies just below consciousness. With awareness, your client can then work more effectively with you in therapy to address the actual issues that are bothering them.

3. **Quieting negative thoughts (Chapter 5):** People who struggle with eating issues often suffer from negative thoughts, perceptions, and self-talk. These thoughts and their internal negative voice contribute to the challenges in mood, self-perception, self-esteem, and self-worth. These constant negative thought patterns become debilitating obstacles. Often, your clients will make decisions based on these negative perceptions that can lead to cycles that feel impossible to get out of. They are essentially in an emotionally abusive relationship with themselves. Our clients often will use food behaviors to escape, avoid, or cope with the negative voice, however, this usually backfires, and the negative thoughts become even louder. Therefore, this foundational skill is imperative for eating disorder recovery. If this skill is weak or was never taught it can be a common cause for relapse.

4. **Practicing self-compassion, self-acceptance, and self-care (Chapter 6):** People who struggle with eating issues frequently resist learning this skill, not because they don't want to but because they don't feel deserving of these basic practices. Our clients feel awkward and uncomfortable, and these practices feel foreign to them. Their negative thoughts can be triggered as they struggle to practice these helpful behaviors (Chapter 5), and they avoid the very tools that would help them. Our clients need to develop this essential skill to get through tough times and recover fully from their eating disorder.

5. **Exploring body neutrality and acceptance (Chapter 7):** Body dissatisfaction is often a challenge for many struggling with eating issues. Cultural messages about body image ideals heavily influence our values and beliefs about what is desirable and admired. When your client is battling with their identity and their self-perception, they can easily believe these misconceptions in order to feel appreciated and respected by others. Through the language of metaphor (Chapter 4), your clients will learn to recognize and identify the meaning behind their true dissatisfaction, rather than focus on surface distraction. They will be able to view their bodies in a neutral way and learn that their dissatisfaction is not really about their body.

6. **Understanding myself in relation to others (Chapter 8):** Research has shown that people who have problematic eating patterns also face issues with social interactions, consistently deal with higher levels of attachment insecurity, and usually exhibit a nonassertive, submissive, interpersonal interaction style with socially avoidant behaviors. Your client may not realize that some of their behaviors can sabotage their ability to develop healthier relationships. This foundational skill emphasizes your client's exploration into understanding their own attachment style and needs, thereby understanding how to interact in relationships. This eliminates the need for them to use other maladaptive coping tools to deal with the disappointments, unmet needs, and other issues that normally arise when in a relationship.

7. **Coping with emotional triggers and building resilience (Chapter 9):** It is imperative for your client to learn how to identify and cope through emotional triggers and emotional distress. Lack of emotional resiliency is one of the biggest predictors of unsustainable eating disorder recovery. Clients must learn various techniques to deal with life's stressors. It is nearly impossible to achieve full recovery from an eating disorder without mastering this fundamental foundational skill.

8. **Using my authentic voice (Chapter 10):** Your client will likely have challenges around communicating and verbalizing how they feel. They may be conflict avoidant, fear anger from others, rejection, or disappointing others (Chapter 8) and thus have trouble allowing authentic transparency and verbalizing their true feelings, needs, wants, and/or desires. If your client cannot master this foundational skill, they will continue to use maladaptive methods to communicate their needs, wants, or feelings, such as with disordered eating behaviors. This skill is also essential for recovery.

9. **Changing my story (Chapter 11):** Your client may have difficulty believing that there is hope in their situation. They see negative thinking patterns, along with other problematic areas, as evidence that their situation can never get better. These beliefs become your client's story. Often their rigid thinking and learned helplessness becomes the structure of their story. Their identity becomes part of this story. Therefore, in order for your client to achieve full lasting eating disorder recovery, they must learn this foundational skill. They must learn to clarify and let go of outdated stories that have become obstacles for their growth and to change their perspective and old beliefs. Your client will learn to create a new story and new beliefs about who they are, so that they can find purpose, meaning, and a recovery story that will lead them to a life free from their eating disorder.

Teaching these foundational skills is imperative for your client's recovery. Your clients will learn to use these essential tools at the start of the recovery process because this will help them stay grounded and empowered. As their recovery progresses, your client will recognize that they will be consistently using these skills. They will notice how the use of the foundational tools becomes more intuitive, natural, and automatic. Gaining awareness about what's fueling their eating disorder is essential for the third step in their recovery process.

As your client's recovery progresses, they will start to use foundational skills to replace the function of their eating disorder. For example, when your client is at the point of awareness where they know exactly why they are using their eating disorder they will be able to identify the function for the behavior, they will be able to choose another more effective skill, eventually replacing their eating disorder. More on this topic as we get to the revealing the function of your eating disorder.

Part 2: Creating Awareness about Underlying Issues through Decoding Metaphors

While decoding food and food behaviors is a foundational skill crucial to your client's recovery, decoding metaphors in general is a big part of working with eating disorders. Chapter 4 is dedicated to understanding the role of metaphor in food and eating behaviors, but it is certainly not limited to that chapter; decoding metaphors will be ongoing work that crosses many domains.

In other words, we have to be aware that whenever our client is struggling with food, body dissatisfaction, food behaviors, or anything to do with their eating disorder, there is something else under the surface that they are having difficulty with. Once you're able to help your client with this, you'll see the difference in your client's progress with food, food behaviors, and their feelings regarding their body.

To uncover what the food represents and to discover the functions of the eating disorder, your goals will be 1) to help bring insight and awareness about unconscious aspects of the eating disorder, 2) to boost the ability to recognize repetitive, pervasive, and entrenched patterns of relating to others, 3) to focus on the dynamics of relationships, and 4) to focus on the expression of affect, and an examination of wishes, fantasies, and core conflicts. This approach mainly focuses on understanding individuals' motives and feelings.

Let's continue to examine the case of Nicole, 19 from Chapter 1, to see how unlikely it is that clients will be able to clearly point out and articulate issues out of their awareness.

Therapist: *"Please say more about getting sick and throwing up, how often does this happen and when did you first notice that this has been a problem?"*

Nicole: *"It's been an issue for as long as I can remember. I started getting sick a lot around age nine. I usually feel queasy and throw up. I don't know if it happened before that, but I know for sure that I started throwing up then because it first happened on my ninth birthday. I usually feel better after I throw up, so sometimes after eating, if I feel too full or ate just a little more than I meant to eat, I might get rid of some of it to feel better. It didn't start out about losing weight but now that I'm eating so much and getting bigger, I found that losing weight is a good side effect. I'm mostly really throwing up because I feel sick, and I always feel better after I throw up."*

Therapist: *"Can you say more about what was going on in your family at nine years old?"*

Nicole: *"Not much. I can't really recall except, that's when my dad moved into the house with us. My mom was a single mom until Dad moved back in when I turned nine. We had the birthday party a few days after he moved in because it was his idea to do the birthday party."*

Therapist: *"Tell me more about your relationship with your mom and dad?"*

Nicole: "Well, as an adult its ok, but that's just because I don't live with them anymore. I moved out of my house as soon as I graduated from high school because I didn't like it there. I don't see them often but when I do, I always have to prepare myself. I feel like I can't stop eating when I go to my mom's. I eat and eat and eat, until I'm so full and hate myself."

Therapist: "How would you describe your relationship with your mom and dad?"

Nicole: "I don't like saying it, but I don't respect her that much. My dad is like furniture to me. He exists and takes up space and I don't know how to feel about him. My dad's like furniture cause he came into my life at nine years old and all he does is works and drinks a case of beer and passes out. Yes, he's an alcoholic. That's why I don't respect my mom. She's so afraid he'll leave her again, so she does whatever he wants. It's gross. It's makes me sick just thinking about it.

             At around age nine, my father came back into our lives. Just out of the blue, this man came to live with us, and I was told that he was my father. It was strange at first since I didn't know him at all, but just like that my mom snapped out of her depression."

Therapist: "Sounds like you didn't have much of a relationship with your father and sounds like you may have some feelings towards your mom?"

Nicole: "I guess. I don't know. I don't care about them. Why should I care about how my mom feels? She always told me that no one would love me. She told me she felt the same way with my dad and that's why she decided to take him back. He put us in a lot of danger so I don't know why she would even take him back, but I guess that's just the way it is."

Therapist: "How did you feel that your mom took your dad back after he put you in danger?"

Nicole: "Ugh, I don't know. I just feel so sick talking about this now. I want to just throw up."

Therapist: "We were talking about your boyfriend earlier in the session and you talked about feeling sick and wanting to throw up. How do you feel this is similar to the way you felt earlier?"

Nicole: "I don't know." (long pause)

Therapist: "Take your time. What are you noticing in your body?"

Nicole: "I don't know. I feel queasy but also really tense and tight, like I can't breathe and want to yell and scream and throw up. I feel like I want to explode!"

Therapist: "That's a lot of intensity you're feeling. I'm wondering if you're feeling anger and when you feel anger like this, you feel like you want to throw up?"

Nicole.   "Yes! I'm so pissed! I'm so pissed!" (sobbing)

Therapist: "Yes, I can see how upset you are. What happens when you share your anger with others?"

Nicole: (still sobbing) "I've never shared my anger with anyone. I just keep it in."

Nicole entered therapy because of the breakup of her two-year relationship. However, in learning more about Nicole and collecting data from her BASIC I.D., it's obvious that there's much more below the surface. Clearly, Nicole is struggling with maladaptive food behaviors, but she isn't aware of how her purging is connected to her feelings. In this example, the purging behaviors is a way for Nicole to get rid of her angry feelings so that she can avoid thinking, feeling, or dealing with the issues that provoke her anger. Anger is uncomfortable for Nicole and it literally makes her feel sick. This is an indication that Nicole has a low tolerance for distress and doesn't know how to cope with intolerable feelings. She "purges" her feelings to avoid having to face the trials and tribulations. From this information we know she needs help with foundational skill *#7 Coping with emotional triggers and building resilience.*

We have learned that Nicole is an adult child of an alcoholic. Her childhood was difficult and unsupportive, and she was emotionally neglected. From this information alone, we know that Nicole needs assistance in developing foundational skill *#6 Understanding myself in relation to others* so that she will be emotionally prepared to work on the deeper issues that will be revealed as psychotherapy progresses. But while all foundational skills are essential from the multimodal perspective, Nicole would likely benefit most with first learning foundational skill *#7 Coping with emotional triggers and building resilience.*

As you work with your clients, you will notice that these metaphors can be found in many areas; you'll be able to identify them and will also be able to help your clients to understand what the metaphors represent, and how they are related and connected to the functions of their eating disorder.

Part 3: Revealing the Function of the Eating Disorder and Uncovering Underlying Issues below the Surface

There can be many functions for your client's eating disorder. The most common function of eating disorders is for coping with discomfort. It helps your client to avoid having to deal with their agonizing reality. Over time, the unaddressed problems and your client's suppressed feelings have been buried and replaced with distractions (that can become obsessions) that they fixate on: body image, weight, food, diets, and their physical appearance. This can lead to a wide range of emotions: frustration, anger, sadness, excitement, envy, jealousy, shame, and guilt. The distractions that your client may fixate on and obsess over are now the identified problems.

The various functions of disordered eating are unique to each individual's circumstance. However, they can also fan across domains. The synergistic effects that each of the domains have on one another can be unbearable. Let's take a look at how disordered eating and related behaviors function for our case example, Nicole. Imagine this occurring in session with Nicole. Below are case conceptualizations of various starting points from all modalities. The function of the eating disorder is highlighted, along with foundational skills and the underlying issues and starting point ideas for therapists to use from each situation.

Behavioral

Nicole had been purging since the age of nine. She stated, "I feel so sick that I just throw up sometimes." However, over the years, the purging behaviors progressed into binge and purge cycles leaving Nicole feeling helpless, "I just can't take the feeling of having food in my body. The last few months, I try to restrict food because I'm afraid that once I start eating, I can't stop. I normally restrict food all day and end up out of control at night. I didn't think it was a problem because I didn't think it was that bad, but now I'm so hungry at night because I don't let myself eat during the day. I eat and eat and can't stop until I'm in so much pain. I can't sleep afterwards because my body feels dirty, unclean and uncomfortable. I end up throwing it up. I make myself throw up until I get everything out. I'll usually take a few laxatives before bed to make sure it's all out. I'm usually sick the next day. I always have bad cramps from the laxatives and when it's all out of me, I feel lighter, emptier and cleaner."

Nicole engages in this behavior daily and has realized that she can't continue to live her life in this way. Her partner recently ended their relationship and so she decided to seek help. She felt that no one would want to be in a committed relationship with her and she felt disgusted and shameful about her actions.

After being in therapy for about nine months, Nicole started to recall feeling "dirty" and "unclean." She hadn't received any previous therapy around trauma or sexual abuse and wonders whether or not she pushed any memories of sexual trauma away. She realized that when she ate she felt more connected to her body and therefore noticed the feelings of shame. Restriction helps her to disconnect and numb from her body. However, because she was restricting food, she was physically starved, and therefore felt out of control when she ate.

This process causes Nicole to binge eat. Binge eating also helps Nicole stay disconnected from her body and to soothe herself. When Nicole felt uncomfortably full, she felt disgusted, shameful, dirty, and unclean. Inducing vomiting and using laxatives to rid the food helped Nicole feel that she had some control over the intolerable emotions and fears that she may have suppressed memories of sexual abuse. These behaviors helped Nicole cope and disconnect from her body so that she could avoid experiencing the "shame" and feeling "dirty."

FUNCTION FOR EATING DISORDER

- *Disconnect from her body to avoid feeling "shame and dirty."*

FOUNDATIONAL SKILLS TO FOCUS ON FOR THIS EXAMPLE

- *#1 Establishing a Mind-Body Connection.*
- *#7 Coping with Emotional Triggers and Building Resilience.*
- *#4 Practicing Self-compassion, Self-Acceptance, and Self-Care.*

UNDERLYING ISSUES TO EXPLORE/ADDRESS

- *"Feeling dirty and unclean" possible unaddressed sexual abuse.*
- *Recent break up with boyfriend.*

Starting point tip:

- Help Nicole understand how the uncomfortable physical sensations she is feeling are not necessarily connected to physical fullness but to emotional fullness.
- Rule out sexual abuse and prepare to refer Nicole to a therapist that specializes in trauma if you do not have the expertise in this area.
- Address the importance of emotional distress tolerance and reviewing tools that help Nicole to stay present and grounded.
- Help Nicole understand the importance of self-care and reviewing realistic tools that she can practice in between sessions.

Affect/Emotional:

Nicole struggles with anxiety and often purges to calm herself. She has difficulty recognizing and acknowledging her feelings.

> *"My family was not very emotional. We were taught in our family that when you show any feelings, you're not in control. I guess my dad learned that from his family since they're all uncomfortable with emotions and no one ever talks about feelings. I remember telling him that I was angry as a kid and he told me, I was wrong for being angry. Sometimes I get anxious or I feel unsettled. I'm not quite sure what the feeling is when things get too much. It's hard for me to be around tension and when situations feel out of control. I feel like it's too much and usually, I feel calmer after I throw up."*

After almost a year in therapy Nicole realized how and why her feelings and emotions have been unbearable and after working through some of it she began to make associations about the origins of the deeper issues that continue to affect her. Therefore, helping clients learn distress tolerance skills is imperative to fully recover from difficulties with eating. But in order to learn how to tolerate discomfort, clients first have to be able to recognize that they are experiencing distress in the first place. Many clients have become accustomed to their anxiety. They experience at least some form of mild discomfort daily. Therefore, their normal emotional baseline is heightened and so they use food behaviors to help bring it down.

FUNCTION FOR EATING DISORDERS

- *Distress and emotional tolerance.*
- *Numbing, avoidance of feelings.*

FOUNDATIONAL SKILLS TO PRACTICE

- *#7 Coping with Emotional Triggers and Building Resilience.*
- *#8 Using My Authentic Voice.*
- *#6 Understanding Myself in Relation to Others.*

UNDERLYING ISSUES TO EXPLORE/ADDRESS

- *Family dynamics.*
- *Feeling out of control (anxiety).*

Sensing/Physical Sensations

Nicole started to connect with her physical sensations after being in therapy for nine months: she began to notice the connection between the physical sensations in her body and what was happening in her environment. Nicole acknowledged that she tried to tune out connecting to her intuition and her "gut feelings." She recognized that these physical sensations felt like a "knowing" in her body, and literally made her sick. She couldn't tolerate the forewarning that her body would give her. She felt these signals and dreaded knowing that she would have to endure what comes with her father's drunkenness.

After nine months of therapy Nicole stated in session: *"I just literally get sick whenever we talk about my dad. I don't know why it makes me feel sick. I feel like I have a stomach ache and feel like I have to go to the bathroom or throw up."*

FUNCTION FOR EATING DISORDER

- *Disconnect from uncomfortable physical sensations (gut feelings, intuition, uncomfortable experiences, memories stored in the body).*

FOUNDATIONAL SKILLS TO PRACTICE

- *#1 Establishing a Mind-Body Connection.*
- *#7 Coping with Emotional Triggers and Building Resilience.*
- *#6 Understanding Self in Relation to Others.*

UNDERLYING ISSUES TO ADDRESS

- *Relationship with father.*
- *Possible victim of childhood abuse.*

Imagery

"When I hear my dad's hard forceful footsteps shuffling on the wooden floors, my mind goes immediately into imagining how drunk he probably is. I'm lying down in my bed, trying to close my eyes and ignore the noises that he makes, but my mind can't help but imagine what he'll do next. Will I see him enter my room?"

As you can see in this example, Nicole's imagination is triggered by her father's drunken movements. She feels literally sick when this triggers traumatic memories of her father lying in bed with her. However, Nicole struggles to understand why she feels like this because she can't recall much except for the fact that her father passes out in her bed. She also knows that she literally feels sick when she hears his movements and when she starts to imagine what might happen next. This example is potentially insinuating that there could be unexplored sexual trauma that Nicole experienced but may have no memory of. The therapist working with Nicole would then explore this area of possible trauma with Nicole when she is ready.

FUNCTION FOR EATING DISORDER

- *Distraction: Nicole's focus on food keeps her distracted from the stimulus of hearing her father's footsteps and what it brings up in her body.*
- *Coping: Nicole feels sick to her stomach when she hears her father's footsteps, therefore, the purging behaviors also help her release some of the anxiety she experiences and also helps her disconnect from being present.*

FOUNDATIONAL SKILLS TO PRACTICE

- *#7 Coping with Emotional Triggers and Building Resilience.*
- *#8 Using My Authentic Voice.*
- *#6 Understanding Myself in Relation to Others.*

UNDERLYING ISSUES TO ADDRESS

- *Family dynamics.*
- *Possible history of trauma/abuse.*

Starting point tip:

- Help Nicole understand how eating disorder behaviors have been her way of coping with disturbing images and experiences.
- Help Nicole to articulate her emotions and needs.
- Continue to work on grounding skills and distress tolerance techniques.
- Refer to therapist specializing in treatment of trauma.

Spirituality

Nicole was asked what she would like the goal of therapy to be, and Nicole stated:

"Lately I've been thinking, 'What's the point?' I've always felt like I don't know what to do with my life. Things got better when I met Brandon, my boyfriend. I felt like I had some hope, you know. We did things together and I felt like I wanted to start my day. It's like I had a reason to be here. I had someone that was at least a friend and that I love and had fun with. Now, I'm so sad. I feel all alone with no one. I don't even know who I am anymore. I have this story in my head that I don't deserve anything good. I thought maybe things would change for the better when I left my parents' house, but it didn't. Things are just as hard. I don't know what I'm supposed to be doing or what I need to do next? I have no clue and I don't even know what I want for myself. I feel so lost."

FUNCTION OF EATING DISORDER

- *Distract from feeling alone and hopeless.*
- *Coping through uncomfortable feelings.*

FOUNDATIONAL SKILLS TO PRACTICE

- *#7 Coping with Emotional Triggers and Building Resilience.*
- *#6 Practicing Self-Compassion, Self-Acceptance, and Self-Care.*
- *#9 Changing My Story.*

UNDERLYING ISSUES TO ADDRESS

- *Self-identity, passion.*
- *Meaning and purpose.*

Starting point tip:

- Focus on more immediate goals such as one for the session or for the week.
- Ask Nicole to share an experience or time where she felt more comfortable with who she is.
- What are some things that Nicole is naturally drawn to?

Cognitive

Nicole struggles with negative thoughts about herself.

> *"I first started comparing myself to others in middle school. I felt like everyone else was prettier, smarter and had more friends than me. I never felt like I was good enough to be with kids my age and didn't feel like I mattered to anyone. I've heard my mom say the same. If she were more attractive, then maybe someone would have married her and she wouldn't have had to be doing it by herself."*

Nicole has internalized her mother's negative statements and they are part of Nicole's negative self-talk, dominating Nicole's negative thought patterns.

At the intake appointment, Nicole had difficulty concentrating and recalling information. She was focused on the immediate issue, the breakup with her boyfriend. She had difficulty focusing on the intake questions, and was distracted by her urges to throw up, complaining about feeling physically sick.

> *"I had a hard time focusing I was fasting and hadn't eaten anything for a few days. I just felt weak and exhausted."*

Nicole had difficulty remembering questions asked and had difficulty tracking and following the intake questions. At first it appeared that Nicole was distraught from the break-up, but it was clear that Nicole was also struggling from intense negative thought patterns. Nicole stated,

> *"My mom was right. She said no one would ever love me. Why would he love someone like me? He could've been with others that were a lot smaller than me. I don't know what I was thinking. Look at me, I'm just gullible and stupid. I don't know if I will ever find love. I didn't think he really loved me anyway. Why would he?"*

People who struggle with eating are more likely to experience self-esteem, self-worth, and sense of self issues. These issues can be influenced by negative childhood experiences at home and in their social environment. As you can see, the cognitive domain is affected by the eating disorder and is a direct result of utilizing food behaviors and also cause her to use these behaviors as an attempt to shut down the thoughts and to escape these thoughts altogether.

FUNCTION OF EATING DISORDER

- *Self-punishment.*
- *Distract from the negative thoughts.*

FOUNDATIONAL SKILLS TO PRACTICE

- *#3 Quieting Negative Thoughts.*
- *#4 Practicing Self-Compassion, Self-Acceptance, and Self-Care.*
- *#9 Changing My Story.*

UNDERLYING ISSUES TO ADDRESS

- *Self-worth issues related to relationship/attachment with mother.*
- *Rejection and abandonment from others.*
- *Negative self-perception self-worth.*

Starting point tip:

- Help Nicole gain awareness about her self-talk and negative thoughts and understand how these cognitions affect her eating behaviors.
- Introduce the concept of self-compassion and identify realistic activities that Nicole can practice for caring for herself.

Note: Expressing self-compassion is often challenging for clients exhibiting such strong negative cognitions. Chapters 5 and 6 will go into more depth about how to work with these obstacles.

Interpersonal

"I have a hard time telling others how I feel or if I don't like something. I'm afraid that if I do tell them how I feel that it won't be okay. They won't like what I have to say. I stopped letting my mom know how I feel about our situation at home because it doesn't really matter what I feel. I guess I didn't really talk to my boyfriend about the things that bothered me because I was afraid that he wouldn't like me. I realize now I may have pushed him away now by always accusing him of not really wanting to be with me."

FUNCTION FOR EATING DISORDER

- *Communication or lack of: Disordered eating behaviors functions as a way to express feelings.*
- *Distraction and coping: Distracting through uncomfortable feelings.*

FOUNDATIONAL SKILLS TO PRACTICE

- *#7 Coping with Emotional Triggers and Building Resilience.*
- *#6 Understanding Myself in Relation to Others.*
- *#8 Using My Authentic Voice.*

UNDERLYING ISSUES TO ADDRESS

- *Fear of rejection and abandonment (issues in related to attachment).*
- *Feelings of unworthiness.*

Starting point tip:

- Help Nicole understand what she was feeling in these situations.
- Help Nicole understand what she wanted to communicate through these behaviors.

Biological/Neurological

Nicole first noticed her worries as a child. She experienced obsessive thoughts about something bad happening to her mother. She worried about being left and feared being alone. She experienced her anxiety in physical manifestations in the form of stomach aches and headaches.

When asked about her diagnosis with anxiety and depression, Nicole stated,

"I was diagnosed with anxiety and depression when I was 18. My doctor prescribed me some antidepressants and some anxiety medications that I'm to take when my anxiety is unbearable. Honestly, I can't tell when my anxiety is unbearable, but realized that my anxiety is pretty bad when I want to throw up. Okay, I haven't been taking my antidepressants because I don't want to have to depend on something like pills you know. I'm scared that I will be dependent on it. That's the last thing I want is to be in the place of needing the medications. Also, I can't help but think that taking antidepressants is weak. I feel like I'm a failure and that something is wrong with me. Also, what if I have to take these pills for the rest of my life?

I don't want to have to take them. I know both my parents and some of their family members have anxiety and depression too. I guess it runs in the family. I just got lucky that I got this from my family and won the lottery that I got the fat genes too. Everyone always says I got the Lewis legs. My calves are big, and I know I got my mom's side of the family's bone structure. It makes me feel awful because my mom always hated her legs too."

Nicole has been dissatisfied with her body shape since puberty.

"I have these legs that have been passed down from Grandma. My mom has it too. This is why I can't wear skinny jeans. If I could just change the way my legs look, I would feel better about myself.

My depression gets so bad sometimes, I don't even want to get out of bed. I feel worthless and just exhausted. I don't have the motivation or energy to go to work."

FUNCTION FOR EATING DISORDER

- *Coping with anxiety and depression.*
- *Distraction by focusing on body dissatisfaction.*

FOUNDATIONAL SKILLS TO PRACTICE

- *#5 Exploring Body Neutrality and Acceptance.*
- *#9 Changing My Story.*
- *#6 Practicing Self-Compassion, Self-Acceptance, and Self-Care.*

UNDERLYING ISSUES TO ADDRESS

- *Anxiety and depression.*
- *Self-acceptance, identity.*

Starting point tip:

- Refer to psychiatrist for medication assessment if Nicole isn't already established with a physician.
- Explore anxiety, depression, and assess suicide risk.
- Identify realistic coping tools that Nicole can practice between sessions when experiencing anxiety and or depression.

Part 4: Using a Multimodality Treatment Approach: Practice and Integrated Process

In the last part of this process, your clients will be utilizing and applying the nine foundational skills in their daily lives. Practicing these essential skills are the most crucial part of the treatment. However, as you know, it can sometimes be challenging and frustrating to convince your client to practice new skills when they've been using methods that gives them immediate relief from their distress.

How do you go about persuading your client to actually apply these skills and continue to utilize them long term?

Key Components for Practicing and Applying Integrated Skills

It is important that after each session, you review with your client the key components that you identified in Part 3 of this treatment process. Over time, your client will be able to recognize these components on their own and will have more incentive to practice these skills because they have a clear understanding of what is happening. This helps your client feel empowered and increases their consciousness in the recovery process. This is essential because often eating disorders are used as a way to cope, or to avoid experiencing uncomfortable feelings when sensing ambiguity, hypocrisy, deceitfulness, manipulation, or when situations don't feel quite right.

Use the following questions to guide and help you to determine your client's treatment goals:

QUESTIONS TO CONSIDER

1. What was the purpose (function) of the eating disorder behavior(s) in the specific situation talked about in session?
2. Which of the specific coping tools do they need to learn? Why? How exactly will these coping tools and skills help? (Identify the foundational skills your client needs to practice from what you learned in the session related specifically to the situation.)
3. What was really going on in the specific situation and what were they trying to avoid? (Name their underlying issue for this specific situation.)

Another necessary step in recovery from an eating disorder is to have your client keep a daily journal to document their feelings, insights, revelations, and experiences when practicing skills. This helps your client practice awareness and reflection about what did and didn't work. This is important because often clients have difficulty staying present and remaining mindful. Your client's journal will need to explore and include the following when practicing techniques.

JOURNAL REFLECTION QUESTIONS AFTER PRACTICING SKILLS

- What happened when I practiced the skill?
- What about this practice made it ineffective for me?
- What do I feel would make it more effective and what am I willing to try?
- Any feelings or insights.

NOTE: All of the foundational skills require some degree of mindfulness. If your client is struggling with the skills it may be because they do not want to be aware and present. They may not realize this until they journal and ask themselves these questions. In this case, your client may require additional resources around specific treatment, such as interventions effective for trauma. If you are not a therapist who works with trauma, then your client will have to be referred to a specialist for this issue.

Further, some clients may make blanket statements such as "I tried all those tools and none of them work for me." These statements often indicate a lack of motivation and shows some resistance towards having to put in effort to practice these skills. When clients make these statements it's highly likely they may not find it beneficial to practice due to past negative experiences.

...**And Remember:** Your client will be practicing the skills in an integrated way. The more your client is able to apply these foundational skills, and recognize what they need, the more your client will recognize how the eating disorder is showing up. Remember, this treatment is not intended to resolve all of your client's underlying issues, although many will be addressed and resolved. The goal of this treatment is for your client to be able to work on the bigger underlying issues by replacing their eating disorder with foundational skills leading to recovery. These foundational skills help our clients deal with what's bothering them without utilizing their eating disorder which is making matters worse.

There are many aspects that need to be considered and can contribute to reinforcing your client's eating disorder. Therefore, there isn't a single approach that can target all aspects. It's necessary to keep the unique individual in mind in order to work through the various areas that are affected. Utilizing various techniques that help your client cultivate and develop the foundational skills are the goals of this approach. Your client's progress determines the effectiveness of each technique. Using the data recorded in your client's journal, you will learn what works best for your client.

Bibliography

Amianto, F. et al. (2017). Naturalistic follow-up of subjects affected with anorexia nervosa 8 years after multimodal treatment: Personality and psychopathology changes and predictors of outcome. *European Psychiatry, 45*, 198–206. doi:10.1016/j.eurpsy.2017.07.012.

De Vos, J. A. et al. (2017). Identifying fundamental criteria for eating disorder recovery: a systematic review and qualitative meta-analysis. *Journal of Eating Disorders, 5*(34). https://doi.org/10.1186/s40337-017-0164-0.

Halmi, K. A. (2005). The multimodal treatment of eating disorders. *World psychiatry: Official Journal of the World Psychiatric Association (WPA), 4*(2), 69–73.

Lazarus, A. A. (1989). *The practice of multimodal therapy: Systematic, comprehensive, and effective psychotherapy.* Johns Hopkins University Press.

Lazarus, C. N. (2019). Multimodal Therapy. In J. Norcross and M. Goldfried (Eds.) *Handbook of Psychotherapy Integration,* Third Edition. Oxford University Press.

Part II

Teaching Mindfulness Skills for Recovery

Chapter 3

Foundational Skill #1
Establishing a Mind-Body Connection

The first foundational skill, *Establishing a Mind-Body Connection*, is essential for eating disorder recovery. Since all other foundational skills build on this skill, this is naturally the first step to helping your client heal from their eating problem. Let's take a look at a case example, Rachel.

> *"I can't tell when I'm hungry or when I'm full. I only notice when I'm either dizzy and faint or when I feel like I'm going to explode. There's no in between for me. I've always been like this. I'm jealous of my friends when they tell me that they had enough and just take a few bites of something. I'm like what the heck, for me that's when I'm trying to diet or cut down on calories. I have no idea what my body is saying. Other times, I think I'm starving but, I just ate. Then I realized I was anxious. It's all confusing."*

Rachel's complaints are consistent with most clients seeking help for eating difficulties. Individuals who have not had any previous treatment for their disordered eating usually have limited awareness about their body cues. This affects their ability to recognize hunger and satiety levels. They have challenges discerning subtle cues, and tend to notice signs only when it's undeniable, as shown Rachel's example.

When your client struggles with recognizing physical bodily sensations, they often confuse what they're feeling for hunger and satiety. When clients are unclear about what they are sensing in their bodies, their anxiety increases—for fear of loss of control. This leads to trepidation about both the process of eating, and of the food itself. Palatable foods become triggers for agitation because your client grapples with temptations that entices them to eat. Your client misdirects their energy into ineffective strategies for eating less and resisting the allure of the food due to the fear of overeating. Your client doesn't realize that they've disconnected from their internal guide which informs them of their hunger and satiety levels.

In order to help your clients reconnect to their bodies and honor their bodies' needs, you will find the following techniques in the chapter presented in the order I found most helpful:

- Identifying distress levels.
- Recognizing emotions and sensations.
- Reconnecting mind and body.
- Differentiating physical and emotional hunger.
- Energy awareness.

This makes sense because the reason your client struggles with eating is because they have disconnected from their bodies to avoid discomfort. They are coping by separating themselves from the pain and distress. In this chapter, the focus is on mind and body connection, using exercises and various techniques to help your client reconnect to their internal processes (physical sensations and emotions). In order to help your client be congruent with their bodies, they will need to be able to detect, recognize, and differentiate what they are experiencing in their bodies in order to address what their bodies' need (Meneguzzo et al. 2022).

DOI: 10.4324/9781032651408-6

What Makes your Client Disconnect from their Bodies?

There are many reasons that people with eating issues may disconnect from their bodies. Understanding the underlying reasons can help you better address specific areas that need to be worked on in therapy. This will give you a good place to start in uncovering the function of their eating disorder.

Let's look at a few reasons for mind and body detachment.

Interoceptive Awareness and Alexithymia

This is your client's awareness of their body signals and all that is happening internally such as hunger, fullness, feeling cold, thirsty, nausea, fast heartbeat, scratchy throat, or feeling feverish. This includes the awareness of your client's inner emotional state. However, studies have shown that people who struggle with disordered eating commonly have difficulties with interoceptive awareness (Brown et al. 2021). This is also commonly associated with alexithymia (difficulty identifying and describing one's emotions), another condition that is commonly found in people who have eating challenges.

When individuals have trouble identifying their emotions, they can easily misinterpret sensations from emotions for hunger or satiety cues (Stevenson et al. 2023.). For example, a perceived vibration in the stomach can be perceived as hunger (such as a growling belly) but may actually be nervousness (the sensation of fluttering butterflies) or excitement.

Because individuals have these impairments, they may have a stronger mistrust of their body than the general population. The strongest connection between impairments in interoceptive awareness and eating disorders symptoms is that individuals do not feel safe in their bodies (Brown et al. 2021). This brings up altered experience, misinterpreting their physical sensations related to hunger and satiety as abnormal and dangerous. This leads your client to mistrust their body's cues—doubting that their body knows what's best. For example, when your client eats a meal, any physical sensation such as fullness, bloating, or tightness in their clothing can be perceived as weight gain or the feeling of "fatness." This reinforces their belief that they cannot trust their bodies. They come to the conclusion, "If I listen to my body, I will surely gain weight."

To better understand how this might be presented in a client, let's take a look at Rachel:

"I don't feel like I can just eat and listen to my body. I don't trust that if I eat, my body will do what it supposed to do. Because the truth is when I eat, I feel like I gained ten pounds, and it's immediate. I feel bloated. My jeans are tighter and I feel super full. How can you tell me that I didn't gain weight because I know I did. I feel fat and it makes me not want to eat. I don't trust my body."

Adverse Childhood Experiences

Individuals who have suffered adverse childhood experiences such as physical, sexual, or emotional abuse have increased rates of body disconnection. Trauma often occurs with dissociation (Yoon et al. 2022.). When people endure these challenges, they may detach from their physical bodies, thoughts, feelings, and memories as a coping mechanism to protect them from distress. Therefore, it is understandable that they would have difficulty noticing hunger and satiety cues.

Food Controlling

This is commonly observed in adolescents and children. Caregivers often monitor the quality and quantity of their children's food (Romano & Heron 2021). This interferes with the individual's ability to tune in to their own bodies' hunger and satiety cues, and they learn to ignore their bodies' needs in order to please the caregiver. With good intentions, we often hear parents say:

- *You need to eat all of your dinner before you get dessert.*
- *There are kids starving, so you need to eat all of your food.*
- *Ok, that's enough for today, I believe you've had enough to eat.*

Food as Rewards

While there is no perfect way of eating, and food is normally used in celebratory ways, if special treats are often given as rewards this can reinforce positive emotions and individuals may be more vulnerable to using food as a way to cope when experiencing negative emotions. This results in eating for emotional reasons rather than following hunger and satiety cues (Meneguzzo et al. 2022). The following are some examples of what you may hear others say:

- *You did so well today, let's celebrate with cake.*
- *If you're able to sit quietly, you get a donut.*
- *Let's get some ice cream, you'll feel better.*

Dieting

When people diet, they are intentionally ignoring their hunger cues in order to restrict food in the hopes of losing weight. Over time, when dieters ignore their bodies' cues, they get to the point where when they are famished, they feel out of control, leading to overeating. They are tempted by external triggers cues such as sight and smell of appetizing foods and often exhibit loss of control rather than focusing inward to cues from their body (Waliłko et al. 2021).

Rumination and repetitive thinking are constantly active in dieting individuals. These thoughts distract the dieter from listening to their body cues and elicit feelings such as guilt or shame as the dieting person responds to their physical needs. Foundational skill *#3 Quieting Negative Thoughts* will be addressed in later chapters.

Now that we have a better understanding why your client may have disconnected from their mind and body, let's begin our work by gauging your client's current baseline of awareness with their mind and body connection.

Identifying Distress Levels

Using the Subjective Units of Distress Scale (SUDS) is a mandatory first step in getting your clients to practice tuning into themselves. Your client may not know or have the words to articulate what they are experiencing, however, they are usually able to discern the various levels of intensity that they are experiencing.

Using the scale helps your client feel less anxious and ambiguous about impressions they experience in their body. This will also enable your client to recognize which coping tools are effective by noticing a reduction in the intensity of distress. Individuals who suffer from disordered eating have a tendency towards instant gratification. When they are experiencing distress, they want to remove the pain instantly, therefore they may give up on effective coping skills prematurely. However, if they are able to recognize that after practicing a coping strategy the discomfort may not have completely disappeared but is noticeably less intense, they will be more inclined to continue to use that tool. This also helps your client learn to tolerate sensations in their body knowing that the intensity of distress is temporary and that it does decrease over time.

CLIENT EXERCISE: SUBJECTIVE UNITS OF DISTRESS SCALE (SUDS)

In this exercise, you will create your own scale to rate the level of intensity of physical sensations or distress you're experiencing.

Objective: To notice what is happening in your body at any given moment.
Directions:

1. For every level on the distress scale, write a description of how you feel or what you tend to do when experiencing that level of distress. Identify the sensations and emotions if you are able to recognize what they are.
2. Remember that this is a subjective scale so the goal here is to just notice what you're feeling and doing internally. There are no right or wrong answers.
3. As you refer back to this scale at various times in your day, notice that the level of intensity fluctuates over time and in various situations.
4. Use Rachel's completed example as a guide.

Rachel's completed example looked like this:

Subjective Units of Distress Scale

   0 – **Totally relaxed**: *I feel calm, and just content.*

   1 – **Concentrating well**: *I can read and write with comprehension*

   2 – **Minimal intensity**: *I feel fine, I can do normal things.*

   3 – **Mild intensity**: *I may not notice anything but maybe a little distracted.*

   4 – **Mild to moderate intensity**: *I'm easily distracted and having harder time focusing.*

5–6   **Moderate intensity**: *Thinking about using eating behaviors.*

   7 – **Moderate to high intensity**: *Intense obsessive thoughts about food.*

   8 – **High intensity**: *Waiting for others to leave to binge on food.*

   9 – **Very high intensity**: *Binging. Extremely irritable, and shame.*

  10 – **Highest intensity**: *Non-stop binging.*

Subjective Units of Distress Scale

   0 – **Totally relaxed.**

   1 – **Concentrating well:**

   2 – **Minimal intensity:**

   3 – **Mild intensity:**

   4 – **Mild to moderate intensity:**

5–6   **Moderate intensity:** (Noticing eating disorder thoughts, but can continue to function

   7 – **Moderate to high intensity**: (Difficulty in staying present, obsessive eating disorder thoughts)

   8 – **High intensity**: (Planning to use eating disorder behaviors)

   9 – **Very high intensity**: (Intense urges to use disordered eating behaviors)

  10 – **Highest intensity**: (Intolerable and engaging in disordered eating behaviors)

Recognizing Emotions and Sensations

Now that your client has an idea about gauging the intensity of their sensations, we need to help them to learn and identify their physical sensations and emotions by teaching specific language. Words helps your client have a better understanding and interpret ambiguous sensations. It helps ease anxiety and enables them to question what might be happening, for example, if your client notices a pulsating sensation in their neck and recognizes that in combination with a heated sensation in their face that feels like anger, they can then ask themselves, "What might I be angry about?" This will help them to take notice of what's happening internally and connect to their current situation.

Often individuals who have eating difficulties also struggle with alexithymia. They struggle to know what they feel or recognize the sensations in their body. If your client is unable to describe and connect to these emotions, then it will be challenging for your client to be able to differentiate these emotional sensations from hunger and fullness. Therefore, while the exercises may seem simple, it is important because it helps the client and the therapist establish a baseline of how connected their clients are to their bodies at the start of therapy. This helps them to know what they need to work on. This exercise also helps your client pay attention to their bodies when certain situations elicit specific physical sensations. For example, Rachel said:

"I had this icky feeling about my sister. I avoided the feeling but had no idea what I was feeling. I realized later the icky feeling was jealousy. I was jealous of what my sister accomplished. I wanted to be successful too."

Rachel didn't know she was experiencing jealousy. She was judgmental about any negative feelings associated with her sister and was confused because she felt supportive of her sister and therefore questioned how she could feel jealousy towards her. When Rachel realized that her jealousy had to do with her own desire to be successful, rather than anything negative towards her sister, she was able to embrace the feeling with less judgment and accept that her jealousy was just information about herself. She was then able identify goals to help her feel successful.

Let's get a baseline with how connected your clients are with recognizing their emotions and how it may manifest in their body.

RACHEL'S WORKSHEET: RECOGNIZING EMOTIONS IN YOUR BODY

Have you ever noticed that emotions show up in your body? For instance, if you're nervous your palms get sweaty. Let's explore how other feelings manifest in your body.

Objective: To become aware of how certain emotions show up in your body.
Directions: Refer to the Feelings List and Body Sensations List to describe how you experience the following emotions in your body.

What sensations do you notice? What do you feel in your body? What thoughts do you notice?

Aches in my lower back, tightness in my shoulders and neck. I don't have any thoughts right now.

Fear: *I usually feel queasy in my stomach, and my thoughts race.*
Anger: *My heart races, and I can't stop thinking about what is angering me.*
Guilt: *I feel an uneasiness in my chest and can't stop thinking about what I did.*
Shame: *I feel like disappearing. I feel icky and like I wish I wasn't here.*
Jealousy: *I feel bitter and resentful and angry at myself.*

Notice any similarities or differences in the emotions and or hunger/fullness sensations experienced. What did you notice? *I tend to eat anytime I feel anything in my body.*

CLIENT WORKSHEET: RECOGNIZING EMOTIONS IN YOUR BODY

Have you ever noticed that emotions show up in your body? For instance, if you're nervous your palms might get sweaty. Let's explore how other feelings manifest in your body?

Objective: To become aware of how certain emotions show up in your body.

Directions: Refer to the Feelings List and Body Sensations List to describe how you experience the following emotions in your body.

What sensations do you notice? What do you feel in your body? What thoughts do you notice?

1. Fear

2. Anger

3. Guilt

4. Shame

5. Jealousy

6. Notice any similarities or differences in the emotions and or hunger/fullness sensations experienced. What did you notice?

CLIENT TOOL: FEELINGS LIST

We can experience dozens of different emotions. But most people rarely stop to assess the nuances of what they're feeling. This list can help you pinpoint what you're feeling right now.

Accepting	Angry	Connected	Disconnected	Stressed
Calm	Agitated	Accepting	Aloof	Anxious
Centered	Aggravated	Affectionate	Numb	Burned out
Content	Bitter	Caring	Bored	Cranky
Fulfilled	Contempt	Compassion	Confused	Depleted
Patient	Cynical	Empathy	Distant	Exhausted
Peaceful	Disdain	Fulfilled	Dissociated	Frazzled
Present	Disturbed	Present	Empty	Overwhelmed
Relaxed	Edgy	Safe	Indifferent	Rattled
Trusting	Frustrated	Warm	Isolated	Rejecting
	Furious	Worthy	Lethargic	Restless
	Grouchy		Listless	Shaken
	Irritated		Removed	Tight
	Moody		Uneasy	Weary
			Withdrawn	

Vitality	Courageous	Despairing	Ashamed	Doubtful
Amazed	Adventurous	Anguish	Bad	Apprehensive
Awe	Brave	Depressed	Humiliated	Concerned
Bliss	Capable	Despondent	Mortified	Dissatisfied
Delighted	Confident	Disappointed	Self-conscious	Disturbed
Eager	Daring	Discouraged	Useless	Perplexed
Ecstatic	Determined	Forlorn	Weak	Questioning
Enchanted	Free	Gloomy		Hesitant
Energized	Grounded	Grief		Reluctant
Engaged	Persistent	Heartbroken		Shocked
Enthusiastic	Proud	Hopeless		Skeptical
Excited	Strong	Lonely		Suspicious
Free	Tenacious	Longing		Ungrounded
Happy	Worthy	Melancholy		Unsure
Inspired	Determined	Sadness		Worried
Invigorated	Valiant	Sorrow		
Lively		Teary		
Passionate		Unhappy		
Playful				
Fearful	**Powerless**	**Tender**	**Hopeful**	**Guilty**
Afraid	Impotent	Calm	Encouraged	Regret
Anxious	Incapable	Caring	Expectant	Remorseful
Nervous	Resigned	Loving	Optimistic	Sorry
Panic	Trapped	Reflective	Trusting	
Terrified	Victimized	Self-loving		
Scared		Serene		
Worried		Vulnerable		
		Warm		

CLIENT TOOL: BODY SENSATIONS LIST

We can experience dozens of different sensations in our body. But most of the time we don't stop to really determine the nuances of what we're feeling. This list can help you pinpoint what you're experiencing right now.

Achy	Dizzy	Gentle
Airy	Drained	Hard
Blocked	Dull	Heavy
Breathless	Electric	Hollow
Bruised	Empty	Hot
Burning	Expanded	Icy
Clammy	Flowing	Itchy
Clenched	Fluid	Jumpy
Cold	Fluttery	Knotted
Constricted	Frozen	Light
Contained	Full	Loose
Contracted	Feverish	

Nauseous	Releasing	Sweaty
Numb	Rigid	Tender
Pain	Sensitive	Tense
Pounding	Settled	Throbbing
Prickly	Shaky	Tight
Pulsing	Shivery	Tingling
Queasy	Slow	Trembly
Radiating	Smooth	Twitchy
Relaxed	Soft	Vibrating
	Sore	Warm
	Spacey	Wobbly
	Spacious	Wooden
	Sparkly	
	Stiff	
	Suffocated	

Reconnecting Mind and Body

Now that you have a baseline of how your client is connected to their body, the next exercise are questions that your client can practice asking themselves when they are noticing sensations in their body to help your client increase awareness and connection to their body and their emotions.

RACHEL'S WORKSHEET: MIND AND BODY CONNECTION

It can feel uncomfortable or even a little scary when your body has a reaction and you're not sure why. Your first instinct may be to get rid of the feeling or ignore it. But likely your body is giving you an important clue about an emotion. Let's find out what it might be.

Objective: To become more aware of your strong mind-body connection.

Directions: When you are feeling a change in your body—for example, suddenly feeling very tired—answer the following questions using the Feelings List and Physical Sensation List. Repeat this exercise any time you want to dig deeper into what your body may be telling you.

1. Pause for a moment and check in with yourself to identify the intensity of what you're experiencing internally. At what intensity are you noticing the sensations? *Right now, it's a 6.*

2. Scan your body from head to toe and pay attention to any sensations in your body. Use the Feelings List and Sensations List above to help you describe what you notice. If you're having difficulty noticing anything. (Example: How fast is my heart beating? How do my palms feel? What do I feel in my stomach or in my back, neck and shoulders?) *My back, shoulders and neck feel achy and stiff. I feel tight and tense.*

3. Now, pause for a moment and check in with yourself to identify what you might be feeling. Using the Feelings List above, describe what you might be feeling? (If you're having difficulty with identifying the feelings, ask yourself: How do I feel: calm, tense, anxious, excited?) *I feel burned out, stressed out, and overwhelmed.*

CLIENT WORKSHEET: MIND AND BODY CONNECTION

It can feel uncomfortable or even a little scary when your body has a reaction and you're not sure why. Your first instinct may be to want to get rid of the feeling or ignore it. But likely your body is giving you an important clue about an emotion. Let's find out what it might be.

Objective: To become more aware of your strong mind-body connection

Directions: When you are feeling a change in your body—for example, suddenly feeling very tired—answer the following questions using the Feelings List and Physical Sensation List. Repeat this exercise anytime you want to dig deeper into what your body may be telling you.

1. Pause for a moment and check in with yourself to identify the intensity of what you're experiencing internally. At what intensity are you noticing the sensations?

2. Scan your body from head to toe and pay attention to any sensations in your body. Use the Feelings List and Sensations List above to help you describe what you notice. If you're having difficulty noticing anything. (Example: How fast is my heart beating? How do my palms feel? What do I feel in my stomach or in my back, neck and shoulders?)

3. Now, pause for a moment and check in with yourself to identify what you might be feeling. Using the Feelings List above, describe what you might be feeling? (If you're having difficulty with identifying the feelings, ask yourself: How do I feel calm, tense, anxious, excited?)

With practice your clients will become familiar with various sensations in their body, tuning into their bodies and identifying words.

Differentiating Physical Hunger from Emotional Hunger

Clients often struggle to differentiate between physical hunger sensations and emotion related sensations because the sensations can feel similar.

In addition, it is common that when your client discusses their maladaptive eating behaviors, they often have no clue about how they felt before or after they ate. Your client usually only notices obvious signs for hunger, such as a loud growling stomach, or feeling lightheaded and dizzy. It is common that they only notice signs that indicate that they're overly hungry or when they feel extremely uncomfortably full. Therefore, your client needs to learn to recognize hunger and satiation levels in order to be able to differentiate them from emotional hunger.

Your client experiences physiological signs that let them know that they are physically hungry. As you know these signals can be experienced as a growling stomach, thoughts about food, tiredness, poor concentration, lack of energy, and irritability. However, when your client has satiated their physical hunger and there are no physical sensations signaling hunger, then likely, they are experiencing emotional hunger.

This is the urge to eat to replace or fill an emotional need or void. When your client is eating for emotional reasons, no amount of food will be able to satisfy their emotional needs. In this chapter, we will focus on physical hunger and learning to differentiate it from emotional hunger. Chapter 4 is devoted to emotional hunger, foundational skill #2 *Uncovering the Meaning Behind Food and Eating*.

The purpose of the next exercise is to get a baseline of what your client currently perceives as physical hunger and emotional hunger signals. This exercise will give you more information about what your client will need to work on.

RACHEL'S WORKSHEET: PHYSICAL HUNGER V.S. EMOTIONAL HUNGER

What does it feel like when you're *physically* hungry? How about when you're *emotionally* hungry? Sometimes it's hard to tell the difference, especially if you've become used to ignoring your body's hunger and fullness cues. Let's find out what messages you're getting from your body.

Objective: Learn to differentiate between physical hunger and emotional hunger.
Directions: Using the Body Sensations List, please answer the following questions.

---

1. How do you know when you are physically hungry? *I feel hungry all the time. I'm not sure.*

2. What physical sensations do you feel in your body when you are hungry? Where do you feel it in your body? *Usually feel lots of movement in my body. Like tickling or something.*

3. How do you know when you are satiated? What does physical fullness feel like in your body? *Usually feel I'm about to explode. My stomach feels tight.*

4. What physical sensations do you feel in your body when you are overly full? Where do you feel it in your body? *Tightness in my belly and pain in my chest. I can hardly breathe.*

5. How do you know you are emotionally hungry? What does emotional hunger feel like in your body? *Like my mouth is needing something. Like my mouth feels restless.*

6. What thoughts do you notice that go through your mind? *Usually feel upset and ashamed that I'm always hungry.*

7. What emotions or feelings do you notice? *Definitely shame, guilt and sometimes anger.*

8. What are some differences between physical and emotional hunger that you have experienced in your mind and body? *I think emotional hunger feels more intense than physical hunger.*

CLIENT WORKSHEET: PHYSICAL HUNGER VERSUS EMOTIONAL HUNGER

What does it feel like in your body when you're *physically* hungry? How about when you're *emotionally* hungry? Sometimes it's hard to tell the difference, especially if you've become used to ignoring your body's hunger and fullness cues. Let's find out what messages you're getting from your body.

Objective: Learn to differentiate between physical hunger and emotional hunger.
Directions: Using the Body Sensations List, please answer the following questions.

---

1. How do you know when you are physically hungry?

2. What physical sensations do you feel in your body when you are hungry? Where do you feel it in your body?

3. How do you know when you are satiated? What does physical fullness feel like in your body?

4. What physical sensations do you feel in your body when you are overly full? Where do you feel it in your body?

5. How do you know you are emotionally hungry? What does emotional hunger feel like in your body?

6. What thoughts do you notice that go through your mind?

7. What emotions or feelings do you notice?

8. What are some differences between physical and emotional hunger that you have experienced in your mind and body?

Now that your client has gained awareness about the physical sensations they experience internally we can introduce the Hunger and Fullness Scale. This is a tool that your client will use to determine where they are with their physical hunger at any given moment.

This is one of the most important exercises for your clients. This is a basic exercise that your client can practice daily. Eventually, your client's natural ability to detect their physical hunger will be restored.

When your client is past the point of hunger and feels shaky, their body can feel out of control, which makes them vulnerable to overeating. If they consistently ignore their hunger cues, they disengage from their body cues and therefore risk severing the ability to detect their body's needs. Honoring their hunger cues when they notice them is a first step to attuning to their body.

People with disordered eating have difficulty believing that others notice hunger and fullness cues and can honor their bodies without many challenges. Our clients commonly believe that they are not able to accommodate their needs at the first sign of noticing hunger signals. *"I'll be at work, or I won't have food with me so what do I do then?"* Your clients will learn to plan ahead for times when they will not have the freedom to eat when noticing a hunger cue during work hours, or when they are in a class. For example, if your client knows that they will be in a situation that won't allow them to eat, they can plan by eating a meal prior to going to work or packing a snack just to hold them over until the next opportunity to eat.

However, people who have the propensity to be restrictive towards food, especially those that are in recovery from anorexia nervosa, will need to have a more regimented eating schedule—eating according to their dietitian's recommended plan. This is because while they are in recovery, they tend to have no physical hunger signs while simultaneously experiencing physical sensations of fullness (Khalsa et al. 2022). For these clients, the hunger scale can still be used to practice learning new sensations, however they cannot fully rely on their perception of their body's signals just yet. They will need to continue to rely on regularly timed meals paying attention to the quality and quantity of food eaten. They may also be struggling with emotions that are causing them to perceive their body as "physically full," misinterpreting this when they are actually experiencing "emotional fullness." We will dive deeper into this in Chapter 4.

The hunger and fullness scale helps your client pay attention to physical sensations and to discern sensations not related to physical hunger. For example, clients may have difficulty distinguishing anxiety from the physical sensations of hunger. The fluttery feelings in their chest and belly can easily be confused for sensations of hunger, like a growling tummy. Or for others, these fluttery sensations are unpleasant and can cause queasiness and therefore, result in a loss of appetite. This can be challenging for your client to recognize early on in their recovery process.

For example, Let's take a look at Rachel:

Rachel, a pharmaceutical representative noticed the time as she sat in traffic, "Just an hour left before the presentation starts" she thought. As she rehearsed her presentation in her head, taking bites from her doughnut, she observed a tingling heavy sensation in her throat and abdomen that felt like hunger. She continued taking bites when she realized the bakery box was nearly empty. (She had purchased several boxes of pastries for the attendees). The tingling sensation was just as intense as it was before consuming the treats, so confusion set in. She made a mental note to talk about the incident in therapy. Rachel realized after sharing her experience that she misinterpreted her anxiety about the presentation and confused it with sensations for physical hunger.

Let's take a look at the Hunger and Fullness Scale:

CLIENT TOOL: HUNGER AND FULLNESS SCALE

It is important for you to practice checking in with your hunger cues before and after you eat. Start the process by asking, "Where is my physical hunger? Where is it on the hunger scale?"

The lower numbers on the scale reflect physical hunger and the higher numbers represent physical fullness and level 5 represents being neither hungry nor full—you're relaxed, able to focus and concentrate easily. You're encouraged to use this tool before and after each meal to practice awareness and tuning into your body. This will help you to practice honoring your body's needs and reconnecting with your body.

0	1	2	3	4	5	6	7	8	9	10

Hunger and Fullness Scale Rating Key

0: **Starving:** Hunger is consistently ignored. Feels extremely dizzy, faint, or may even have fainted.

1: **Overly hungry:** Feeling lightheaded and dizzy.

2: **Strong hunger:** Clear intense hunger cue, headache, difficulty concentrating, irritability, and growling stomach.

3: **Clear hunger signal:** Subtle but clear hunger signal. Food sounds appealing, thinking about food options. Lightness and obvious hunger signs but not quite uncomfortable. Level 3 is ideal to honor hunger cues.

4: **Subtle hunger**: noticeable light subtle cues, but not quite hungry yet. Food starting to sound appealing.

5: **Neutral/ satisfied:** You're feeling neither full nor hungry. You're easily able to focus and concentrate on the task at hand and feeling content.

6: **Subtle fullness:** You recognize subtle fullness. You experience a lightness in your body. You can have more bites of food since you aren't quite satiated. You're physically comfortable, and mindfully eating. Your food is still enjoyable.

7: **Just full**: Your Body feels balanced. Clear obvious hunger cues have disappeared. You're noticing physical fullness and can take another bite of food and still not feel overly full, but the extra bite is not needed. Ideally, level 7 is where you feel comfortably satiated.

8: **Notch past full**: There is a clear physical indication that you're feeling full, experiencing tightness and discomfort. Continuing to eat can lead to feeling physically uncomfortable and heaviness in your body.

9: **Overfull**: Uncomfortably full and adjusting your clothing, loosening belts, buttons, and buckles. Your body feels stretched and tight, and you're having a challenging time with energy levels, feeling sluggish and heavier in your body.

10: **Uncomfortable and stuffed**: Extremely uncomfortable. You may feel extremely full feel like you may burst. These sensations trigger urges to get rid of the food. You're unable to focus and concentrate on any task. You may notice your critical voice, judgments, or negative self-talk, using harsh and punishing words and may be experiencing tremendous guilt and shame.

CLIENT EXERCISE: HOW PHYSICALLY HUNGRY AM I?

At first using the hunger scale and practicing mindful eating can be challenging, however now that you are aware of the hunger and fullness scale, it is also important to remember that your body is unique and that what you experience may differ from how others experience hunger and fullness sensations. Therefore, pay attention to what your body needs by allowing your mind to freely investigate your experiences with curiosity.

Objective: To learn your body signals and to honor your body's needs.
Directions:

1.   Before and after each meal, check in with your body using the Hunger and Fullness Scale Rating Key.
2.   Use the questions below to check in with your body to determine how physically hungry you are.
3.   Use these questions before every meal in conjunction with other exercises that follow.

1. Where is your physical hunger on the scale?

2. What physical sensations lets you know where you are on the hunger scale?

3. If you are having difficulty determining your physical hunger, check other facts by asking: When was the last time you ate? What did you eat? How much did you eat?

4. Other questions to consider. Ask yourself if anything else might be hindering your ability to connect with yourself, such as intense emotions, or more or less physical exercise than usual, or anything related to your health, such as any illness.

Therapist Tips

• *Your client will eventually be able to recognize their physical hunger. The more they check in with their body, the more information they will receive from their body to help their process of determining their hunger and fullness levels.*
• *Use the hunger/fullness scale to check in with your client during sessions. This will help you quickly assess whether their issue relates to physical hunger or if you need to address deeper issues that contributed to emotional eating or restrictive food behaviors.*

Energy Awareness

Your client may eat for other reasons other than hunger. For example, it is common for clients to ignore other cues such as their body's need for rest. When people are bombarded with deadlines their basic need for rest may be ignored, resulting in your client eating for energy to complete a task.

If your client had paused just for a moment, connected and listened to what their body needs, they may have noticed that their body may just be in need of a break.

When your clients ignore their need for rest and/or sleep, they will tend to eat as a quick energy boost to feel energized. Physical exhaustion can be easily mistaken for hunger. (However people who restrict their food need to honor their physical hunger cues, in order to gain more energy.)

Connecting, listening, and honoring what their bodies need may appear simple. However, it can be complex and confusing. Often, our clients mistakenly believe that their anxiety is related to their overeating and the weight they gained. They may weigh themselves in an effort to control their anxiety. As we all know, people struggling with weight, body image, and food issues have a tendency to use the number on the bathroom scale to determine if and how much they should eat. As we know the bathroom scale affects your client's mood, motivation and, sabotages everything about recovery and body connection.

Therefore, teaching your client to replace the bathroom scale with the hunger and fullness scale and the physical and emotional energy levels scale gives them a measurement they can focus on when they are feeling distress, or to gauge what they are experiencing. These scales will help your client connect to what they are experiencing in their bodies.

Energy levels play a role in your client's vulnerability: individuals don't realize how they have the urge to eat when they are overly tired and in need of rest. Instead of resting, they unconsciously reach for food for energy. The next mindful practice in connecting to their energy levels help them to determine physical hunger and whether your clients are actually using food to ignore their need for sleep and are just in need of a break.

CLIENT EXERCISE: AWARENESS OF PHYSICAL AND EMOTIONAL ENERGY LEVELS

Let's imagine that you're feeling hungry. So you check in with the Hunger and Fullness Scale and you determine that no physical hunger sensation is present. After glancing at the clock, you realize you just had a meal, so you are certain that you are not physically hungry. Yet, you still want to devour something sweet. This would be an opportunity to check in with your energy levels.

Objective: To check in with your energy levels so you can determine what it is that your body really needs.
Directions: Refer to the Physical and Emotional Energy Scale. Then scan your body. Start by bringing awareness
    to the top of your head, then scanning your entire body all the way down to your feet.

Physical Awareness

- Where is your level of physical energy on the scale?
- How do you know that you're experiencing that level of energy?
- How does your body feel? Your back, neck, shoulders?
- How do your eyes feel?
- Do you have enough energy to sprint, run, jog, or walk the dog?
- What physical activities have you engaged in this week, if any?
- What has your sleep and rest been like this week?
- How much self-care have you engaged in?
- What other curious questions can help you determine what your energy levels are?

Identify where your physical energy levels are on the scale. What does your body need?

Physical Awareness
What does it feel like in your heart and in your mind? Does it feel heavy, light, exhausting, clear, overwhelming?

- Where is your emotional energy on the scale?
- What has this day/week been like for you emotionally?
- How are you feeling in your heart and in your mind?
- What has been happening that feels unsettling, heavy or draining?

Identify where your emotional levels are on the scale. What does your body need?

You may notice that your physical and emotional energy levels are similar, or they may be different. It is important to honor your body's needs in both cases.

Locate where you are with your energy levels. If you are feeling physically exhausted, maybe needing to rest, honor your body by taking a break, maybe even taking a nap. When you're physically exhausted and you honor your body with rest you will notice the cravings and urges for food disappear.

When you are struggling to determine where you are on the scale, you can check the facts to give you clues about what you may be experiencing and needing which means asking yourself objective questions to help you increase your awareness. The following questions help you to determine what may be going on:

- What time was your last meal or snack?
- What did you eat?
- How much did you eat?
- What's been going on lately, emotionally, physically?
- How much sleep have you been getting?
- How active have you been?

CLIENT TOOL: THE PHYSICAL AND EMOTIONAL ENERGY SCALE

0	1	2	3	4	5

The lower the number the more physically or emotionally tired you are. The higher the number, the more physical and or emotional energy you have. Number 3 would be considered neutral, not overly tired nor overly energetic.

0: Struggling to stay awake, may feel sick, dizzy, nauseated.

1: Physically or emotionally depleted, exhausted, and/or drained. You may need to rest or take a nap, and likely you have not practiced or engaged in self-care activities.

2: Feeling irritable and unsettled. Your body feels heavy. Likely you haven't had the time to take a break and engage in self-care activities. You may not be getting enough sleep and or relaxation. Your stress levels are increasing.

3: Feeling neutral and grounded. You are not experiencing excessive amounts of energy nor are you feeling sluggish. Self-care activities need to be engaged in regularly to prevent from falling below level 3.

4: Feeling content, focused, and alert. You continue to crave movement and you are emotionally balanced.

5: Feeling energized, alert, focused, your body craves movement and joyful activity, and your mind feels the need for creative stimulation.

What if your client still has challenges with hunger and satiation cues even after practicing identifying sensations using both scales? What if your client doesn't experience any signals at all? This is common. Many people who have ignored their body cues for years have great difficulty when first in recovery noticing any cues. Many are also confused by sensations of any kind and have no idea what they are feeling.

The next exercise helps your client practice mindfulness while eating. Mindful eating is observing, noticing, and experiencing with openness and curiosity. This process can be easily learned and is similar to taking a walk or observing nature. For example, when your client starts to eat, they may ask questions such as: *What am I noticing in my body? Do I like the taste, textures, flavors of this food?*

People who struggle with eating are rarely present and mindful during meals. These days multitasking is the norm, so it's not surprising that your clients may be eating on the go or while working, on the phone, or in front of the television.

The goal here is to help your client notice subtle cues. Eating behaviors serve many functions as detailed in Chapters 1 and 2. Therefore, practicing mindful eating is important because it does the exact opposite of what emotional eating does. Emotional eating is about soothing from discomfort by numbing and avoidance. Mindful eating is about paying attention to subtleties so that the individual can increase their awareness and are therefore present with themselves and all that is going on around them. Initially, this can trigger anxiety resulting in challenges when practicing these exercises. Practicing curiosity helps your client make connections needed to uncover the hidden issues that they have been avoiding.

Not only do clients have struggles with sensing hunger cues, they also tend to have challenges with recognizing satiation cues. Therefore, practicing mindful eating is an important component for recovery. It helps them tune into their stopping point, so that they can stop eating at a comfortable level as opposed to stopping only when the food is gone and when they are uncomfortably full.

CLIENT EXERCISE: MINDFUL EATING

Let's imagine you are having difficulty recognizing hunger cues or various physical sensations. This would be an opportunity for you to practice mindful eating during meals.

Objective: To practice mindful eating and learn your body's hunger and fullness cues.
Directions: Complete the worksheet below while you are doing the mindful eating exercise.

1. What is your goal or intention? (Identifying an intention helps you stay focused. Your goal or intention can be as simple as just sitting without distractions while mindfully eating, or something more challenging, such as practicing identifying specific physical sensations.)

2. Where is your physical hunger on the scale?

3. Notice your food. Notice the colors, textures, aroma and smell of the food while taking bites and pausing in between. What flavors do you like or dislike?

4. What textures do you like or dislike?

5. What sensations tell you to have another bite?

6. What sensations tell you that you need to stop eating?

7. What do you notice in your body?

8. What do you notice in your mind?

Continue this process while connecting and tuning into your body. Take two bites, pause and check in. Take another two bites and check in with what you're experiencing in your body. Continue this process until you recognize a signal alerting you to fullness. This will eventually become second nature for you.

Emotional Hunger

Now that you have introduced mindful eating, your clients will notice that at times they aren't physically hungry or physically exhausted but they still have urges to eat. Therefore, your clients will need to know what do when they have determined that their hunger is emotional.

Some people may decide to get rid of or distract themselves from tempting food. However, because the origin is emotional, the urge to eat when not hungry will return unless the metaphor for the food is decoded and addressed. We will go into how to decode emotional hunger in the next chapter, foundational skill #2 *Uncovering the Meaning Behind Food and Eating*.

Often clients will struggle with negative thoughts and judgments when they experience emotional urges to eat so the next exercise will help your client practice curiosity rather than judgment. They may distract or even eat perceived "healthy foods" as a substitute to avoid feeling guilt for having eaten food that is considered off limits. This causes your client to obsess over the food that they avoided.

CLIENT EXERCISE: EMOTIONAL EATING WITH CURIOSITY

When you've ruled out physical hunger but you still have the urge to eat you're probably on the verge of eating emotionally. Let's bring clarity to what this means for you by trying this exercise the next time you want to reach for food in the absence of physical hunger. It is the first stop on your mindful eating journey.

Objective: To practice mindful and curious eating to discover the meaning behind food and the function it serves.

What you will need:

- Time: 20 minutes.
- Something to eat.
- Journal.
- Pen.

Directions:

1. Complete this exercise when you feel the urge to eat when you're not physically hungry.
2. Grab your journal and pen.
3. Choose something to eat.
4. Sit down where you won't be disturbed and write down the answer to the first question below.
5. Then begin to eat mindfully. Answer the remaining questions as you eat.

1. What is your intention or goal? Write your goal for this exercise at the top of the journal page. The goal of the exercise is to help you stay focused, and it would be beneficial for you to come up with goals specific to your situation. Some examples of goals include:

   • To practice awareness around food specifically when you are not physically hungry.
   • To slow down and find the function of the food.
   • To increase awareness around emotional needs.
   • To investigate what the food is representing.
   • To understand why the food feels overwhelming.
   • To practice finding the metaphor in the food.

2. As you are eating, ask yourself these questions:

   • What about this food makes it so tempting?
   • What does this food remind you of?
   • What does this food promise you right now?
   • What do you feel could change right now if you ate this?
   • What does this food feel and taste like in your mouth?
   • What are you feeling right now as you take bites of this food?
   • What do you notice in your body, mind, and thoughts?

3. Take another bite and pause while asking curious questions, then take another bite while completing the worksheet questions, or recording responses in your journal.

   • What does this food taste like? What do you like most about this food?
   • What's happening to your thoughts as you eat this food mindfully?
   • What are you feeling in your body, mind, and heart?
   • What are some emotions you are able to connect with?
   • What are you enjoying from this food?
   • What is the texture of the food?
   • What are you trying to disconnect from or avoid?

4. Take another bite. Continue eating mindfully while asking yourself questions about why the food feels satisfying for you. Continue this process until you have either no interest in continuing to eat or when you are done eating.

5. Notice what you recorded in your journal about your food. Do you notice any themes? Circle the adjectives that may give you hints about what is going on in your life and is playing out in your food.

The data in your journal provides clues about what may be happening in your life that you may not have had awareness about.

The data will help you decode the metaphor behind the tempting food. This exercise can be used in conjunction with the metaphor exercises found in Chapter 4 which will assist you in uncovering what is happening in your life and highlight the real issues that need to be addressed. Having awareness of the real issues helps remove the power from the food, resulting in food just being food.

When the function for the food is taken away, the distraction of what it represents is no longer there. We are left to deal with the issues that are causing uncomfortable feelings. Let's continue on to Chapter 4, foundational skill *#2 Uncovering the Meaning Behind Food and Eating* to learn to decode food behaviors and learn more about emotional hunger.

Bibliography

Brown, T. A. et al. (2020). Body mistrust bridges interoceptive awareness and eating disorder symptoms. *Journal of Abnormal Psychology, 129*(5), 445–456. https://doi.org/10.1037/abn0000516.

Khalsa, S. S., Berner, L. A., & Anderson, L. M. (2022). Gastrointestinal Interoception in Eating Disorders: Charting a New Path. *Current Psychiatry Reports, 24*(1), 47–60.

Meneguzzo, P., Garolla, A., Bonello, E., & Todisco, P. (2022). Alexithymia, dissociation and emotional regulation in eating disorders: Evidence of improvement through specialized inpatient treatment. *Clinical Psychology & Psychotherapy, 29*(2), 718–724. https://doi.org/10.1002/cpp.2665.

Romano, K. A., & Heron, K. E. (2021). Regulatory parental feeding behaviors, emotion suppression, and emotional eating in the absence of hunger: Examining parent-adolescent dyadic associations. *Appetite, 167*, 105603.

Shank, L. M. et al. (2019). The association between alexithymia and eating behavior in children and adolescents. *Appetite, 142*, 104381. https://doi.org/10.1016/j.appet.2019.104381.

Stevenson, R. J. et al. (2023). The development of interoceptive hunger signals. *Developmental Psychobiology, 65*(2), e22374.

Waliłko, J., Bronowicka, P., He, J., & Brytek-Matera, A. (2021). Dieting and Disinhibited Eating Patterns in Adult Women with Normal Body Weight: Does Rumination Matter? *Nutrients, 13*(7), 2475. https://doi.org/10.3390/nu13072475.

Yoon, C. et al. (2022). Adverse experiences as predictors of maladaptive and adaptive eating: Findings from EAT 2018. *Appetite, 168*, 105737. https://doi.org/10.1016/j.appet.2021.105737.

Chapter 4

Foundational Skill #2

Uncovering the Meaning Behind Food and Eating

One of the many reasons eating disorders are complex to treat is that nearly everything in the world of eating disorders is metaphorical. This means that seemingly innocuous things—for example, a bag of potato chips, eating before bedtime, or the belief that carbs are bad—may be serving as symbols of something entirely different, such as love, an insecure attachment, or a need for control. In other words, eating disorders are not what they appear to be. Let's unpack with this means.

Why is it important for therapists and clients to understand the metaphorical language of eating disorders?

Our emotions, thoughts, feelings, and unconscious processes are communicated from our soul through metaphorical language (Landau 2018). This is where our spiritual yearnings, needs, and desires reside. Through symbols, representations, and art, our soul communicates to us what we need. However, at times we can become confused and interpret the soul message literally (Malkomsen 2021).

To understand this a little better, let's take the phrase, "conscience is a man's compass." We can easily view this quote by Van Gogh metaphorically to mean that we can use our conscience like a moral compass to show us the right path. However, if we take the message literally, we may feel that we need direction and literally use a compass daily to find our way. Our soul may give us clues, but we must interpret and look beneath the surface to really understand what we need (Casasanto & Gijssels 2015).

How many times have our clients been told to either *stop eating* or to *eat more*? If it were that simple, eating disorders would not exist. This tells us the eating disorders are not just about the surface behaviors and what we think is going on. There is more under the surface that your client has no awareness about. The food behaviors, feelings, and emotions related to food are just the tip of the iceberg, and the issues below the surface need to be identified.

This chapter looks at how your client's unconscious processes affect their eating and behaviors, and helps you to teach your clients curiosity by exploring and asking the questions that help them to dig deeper, uncovering their challenges (Thompson-Brenner 2014). This will help your clients gain awareness and become more conscious about their circumstances.

Let's take a look at Albert. At 29 years old, Albert has been struggling with emotional eating for as long as he can remember. He came into therapy due to his binge eating on pastries, which has been a concern since his recent diagnosis with diabetes. Lately, the emotional eating of pastries, specifically chocolate donuts, has been out of control. When asked, about the first time he recalled eating pastries or chocolate donuts, Albert shared the following:

"I was diagnosed with a hearing impairment at age five. My mom and dad fought a lot and eventually my dad moved out and my mom became a single mother. I still think they fought because of me. It was too stressful for them, and I was their burden. My dad moved to another state when I was six years old, and the last thing I heard was that he had passed away when I was 17. I had activities afterschool to give my mom respite since she had no help. Some days I had an audiologist help me with my hearing.

Amy, my afterschool helper, took me to Dunkin' Donuts every day. I always got a donut and chocolate milk. Mom gave Amy $5 to get it for me. She knew how much I hated having to do afterschool activities. I guess Mom thought that the donut would help, and it did. Mom always gave me chocolate cookies and milk at home when I had a bad day. She'd tell me, I love you on your good days and bad. The treats were just like a hug. It did help me feel better and I knew Mom loved me."

DOI: 10.4324/9781032651408-7

In this example, it is clear that the pastries represent Albert's mother's unconditional love and acceptance. When this was discussed in session, Albert said, *"Mom passed away a few years ago. It was hard. I still eat donuts, chocolate cookies and milk and can't seem to stop. Now I see that it's because it reminds me of the unconditional love I got from Mom. I'm scared that I'll be a burden to anyone in my life, like I was to Dad, and don't want to open myself up to someone that way."*

As you can hear in Albert's response, Albert's emotional eating worsened when he lost his mother. He's missing her unconditional love and acceptance and has not completely worked through the emotions that he experienced after his father's abandonment. Albert fears vulnerability in developing relationships due to his fear of rejection and is using food as a way to soothe and comfort himself.

Uncovering the meaning of the food will allow the therapist to help Albert by identifying the underlying issues that have been fueling Albert's urges to binge on these sweets. From just the little information we have been given so far these include:

- A need for unconditional love and acceptance.
- Grief from the loss of his mother.
- Unresolved feelings from abandonment by his father.
- Feelings regarding his disability and being a burden to others.
- Fear of rejection by others.
- Lack of human connection and supportive relationships.

Specific food choices contain valuable information and give us clues about the deeper issues. Our clients tend to judge and punish themselves for having urges or feel guilty engaging in food behaviors and miss the message that their soul is communicating through feelings, sensations, and cravings (Rucińska & Fondelli 2022). Instead, our clients tend to focus on restraining themselves from eating. Then, when they give in, they tend to get distracted by their guilty feelings and the deeper messages are missed.

If Albert avoids his broader feelings (grief over the loss of his mother, for one) and continues to just focus on the shame and guilt he experienced when he eats, he isn't able to recognize the specific function of that particular food. If he is not physically hungry and continues to eat, Albert is eating emotionally. Albert will be able to identify what he needs emotionally by paying attention to his food cravings objectively and compassionately, rather than in a punitive, judgmental way. If Albert is taught curiosity and how to decode the metaphor behind his hunger and what he chooses to eat, it will give him the ability to uncover his soul's hunger.

Eating Disorder Recovery as a Metaphor

Let's look at how one classic movie can symbolize this complex journey of recovery from eating problems. The "The Wizard of Oz" starts out in black and white. Dorothy (client) is upset over threats about having her dog taken by a neighbor (real problem). Dorothy has difficulty dealing with this, so she decides to run away (avoidance of reality). As she runs, a twister touches down (eating behavior). She hits her head (becomes unconscious) and is now in the world of Oz (metaphorical world).

Dorothy (client) is lost and trying to find her way back home (back to her authentic self). She seeks out the wizard (the answer: this is whatever your client thinks will help them feel ok, such as the ideal body) to help her get home (back to her authentic self). The wizard (ideal body) then becomes the answer. If only she gets to the wizard (ideal body), she will be ok. On her journey, she discovers parts of herself that need to be connected in order to help her successfully get home. The parts are: mind/thoughts (scarecrow), feelings/emotions (tinman), and physical body (lion).

On this journey, the witch (fears) follows her and shows up wherever she is and at times so does Glenda (intuition). She reaches what she thinks may be the wizard (ideal body) and is disappointed because it was not what she expected. It wasn't the answer she was looking for. Everything wasn't ok even after finding the wizard (ideal body). She wasn't able to get home (back to authentic self). At the end, through the process, she learns to trust her intuition and discovers what she needed to be ok existed in herself all along and it was revealed through the process of her journey (recovery).

The eating disorder world is much like Oz: you'll learn how to decode food and eating disorder behaviors so that you can help your clients understand what's beneath the food and eating disorder behaviors. Let's get started!

The Family Meal

Our eating processes are heavily influenced by our family experiences. Food rules, food and body image comments, family meals, values, holidays, and family dynamics can contribute to how we unconsciously deal with food. For example, food can be used as a reward, love, punishment, acceptance, rejection, and or support to name just a few. In this way, food serves both as a function and as a metaphor, as you will see in the following exercise.

Memories of having routine meals with our families, holiday gatherings, and/or times where food was used to celebrate helps identify where our beliefs about food originated. Commonly our food experiences as children shapes our behaviors and how we feel about food. This is why a good place to start is getting to know a little about your clients' mealtime routines, specifically during childhood. This allows you to learn about their family system and about their eating rituals, and helps your client reflect on their childhood memories around food, family, and emotions. This helps them understand where some of their beliefs and symbols may have originated.

CLIENT EXERCISE: THE FAMILY MEAL

Can you recall your earlier experiences with food? This exercise can help us discover how earlier experiences contribute to our relationship with food and influence our views and feelings about food in overt and covert ways.

Objective: To gain insight about our earlier experiences with meals, family, and our feelings that may continue to influence us today.

What you will need:

- Time: 60–90 minutes.
- Quiet room or room with calming music (optional).
- Art supplies such as crayons, pastels, markers, drawing pencils.
- Drawing paper.

Directions:

1. Pick a time in your childhood that stands out. A good age to focus on is around seven, which is when people tend to remember. It is also an age when we have awareness of our feelings, of others, and what is happening around us. However, if this age does not feel significant for you, pick whatever age does.
2. Find a comfortable sitting position, with your eyes closed; visualize yourself at the age that you chose to focus on. With your eyes closed ask yourself some of the questions below to help you in your visualization. The visualization should be about 10–15 minutes.

   - Where did I live? Who did I live with?
   - What did our kitchen look like?
   - What did our dining room look like?
   - What was the shape of our dining room table?
   - Were meals home cooked?
   - Where did everyone sit at mealtime?
   - Who was at the table?
   - What was the conversation like during mealtime?
   - What were the unspoken/spoken rules?
   - What were foods that were served? Was it pre-plated, family style, or buffet style?
   - What were the expectations about finishing our food, or desserts, and seconds?
   - What was the mood like during meals?
   - What was the background like, did we have the television on or play any music?
   - What did I recall feeling at mealtime?
   - Were we allowed to have a beverage during meals? What did others have to drink?
   - What time were meals generally?
   - Who helped in the kitchen preparing and cleaning up?

3. After visualizing, draw the details of your visualization. Go through the questions again, this time by illustrating your visualization on your drawing paper. It is important that you do not judge your visualizations, or drawing, instead allow yourself to create without judgment. Give yourself about 45 minutes for this process.

4. Take a look at your drawing and sit with it for a few minutes and notice. Some sample questions you may want to think about are found below:

   - What do I feel looking at this drawing?
   - What did I notice throughout the exercise?
   - What am I feeling?
   - What came up for me that was not expected?
   - What things were known before doing this exercise?
   - What things surprised me about this exercise?
   - What are some patterns and or themes that still exist today?
   - How do the relationships with family affect my thoughts and feelings about food?
   - What new insights do I have about this exercise and my relationship with food?

5. Journal your experience. Using the questions above and adding other important observations, record what you noticed.

6. Share your drawing with your therapist and discuss the process.

Therapist Tips:

- *The "Family Meal" exercise commonly evokes powerful emotions that your client may not have expected. This exercise may also provoke other memories or feelings from childhood that they may have suppressed. Therefore, this exercise is best done in session together.*
- *It's a good idea to allot enough time to debrief/ process feelings and to close the session with a self-care exercise.*
- *Be sure to address/follow up with any memory that brings up significant feelings for your client.*

Here's a case example of Leah who completed the "Family Meal Exercise."

Leah, 45, struggles with restricting food intake. She had been in and out of treatment programs and continues to have difficulty with urges to restrict food. She feels uncomfortable in her body and doesn't like the way her body feels after she's eaten.

Leah completed the Family Meal exercise, which revealed that mealtimes were intense and lonely. Leah drew a round dining room table and depicted empty chairs except for the seat she drew herself in. Leah illustrated food in the microwave and frozen meals in the freezer. Sweets were plentiful and easily accessible throughout her house. Although, she did not recall anyone eating with her, she was clear that her mother shopped for convenient frozen dinners and always gave her microwaved meals. There were no people beside herself in her drawing, just her dog. After completing the exercise, Leah immediately felt heavy and empty at the same time. She was full of emotion and remembered that she only had her dog. "Honestly, I don't even remember anyone taking care of the dog, it wasn't like I was close to the dog. In fact, I don't even know who fed the dog. I can't remember. I just remember it being there. I wasn't a kid that fed it under the table or anything." Reflecting on her family, she realized that her various packaged meals were her only comfort. It was typical for Leah to eat at the empty table with the television on in the background. She didn't recall what programs she would watch on television. "It was just on." Leah's mother struggled with her own undiagnosed mental health issues and was a teenager when she gave birth to Leah.

Leah admitted that for her, eating was her way of just passing time. Food represented comfort and connection for her, and she realized that food was the symbol of love from her mother. Leah loved and resented her mother simultaneously. She felt that her mom sabotaged her eating. Through this exercise, Leah gained insight about the deeper meaning about her food behaviors that reinforced the anger towards her mother.

She said, "I couldn't say no to my mom. In fact, I couldn't share anything with her. I couldn't have feelings because I was supposed to just be grateful for having a mom that took care of me. Mom would always tell me she had it worse because she was a teen mom and would tell me how much she gave up for me. When I was growing up, Mom would be upset and hurt if I didn't eat her microwaved meals. I felt bad and ate it in front of her, even when I wasn't hungry. If I ate, my mom thought that everything was okay, and that nothing was wrong."

Leah's main struggles are restricting food intake. After Leah completed the exercise, she was asked to identify symbols and metaphors that she felt may represent something else. You may want to engage in this type of dialogue with your client by following the example.

Example Script: Post-Family Meal Exercise

Leah:	*"We actually lived with my grandparents during that time, but for some reason I don't remember them being around at meals. They never ate with us. My grandparents lived downstairs of this duplex, and we lived upstairs. I'm pretty sure they were working or something. I never knew my dad. If I have to look for symbols in this drawing, I would think that the empty chairs probably represent something. Also, the microwaved meals and maybe the dog?"*
Therapist:	*"Okay, what do you feel the empty chair may have represented?"*
Leah:	*"A reminder that I'm alone, that no one cares."*
Therapist:	*"How do you feel that affects your struggles with eating today?"*
Leah:	*"Well, I'm not sure if this is it or not but I don't like eating with others. I can't eat around people."*
Therapist:	*"What does microwaved food represent?"*
Leah:	*"Ugh, I hate to say this, but I think maybe my mom since she was the one always pushing food on me and the one making it for me. It also represents how my mom never had time for me and just did things to get by that looked like she cared."*
Therapist:	*"How do you feel that the metaphor about food and your mother affects you today?"*
Leah:	*"Well, I have a love and hate relationship with food. I mostly am afraid of it because I'm afraid I can't control it when I start eating. It's just better to not even deal with it, just don't even start. That's how I feel about my mom. I'd rather not deal with her and her emotions, it's just too much and it's always about her. She still doesn't have the time for me."*
Therapist:	*"Okay, how about the dog? What do you feel the dog represents?"*
Leah:	*"Oh, that's easy. The dog is me."*
Therapist:	*"Tell me more about that."*
Leah:	*"That's how I felt my whole life and even now, like I don't exist. Everyone else has out of control feelings and are demanding about things. I'm supposed to just be there like a dog, alive and breathing with no voice, no needs or wants and just be obedient."*

As you can see with this example, with the help of the therapist Leah was able to identify representations that contained valuable information. From just the symbols, the therapist was able to help Leah gain awareness about the processes that were not in her consciousness. Through identifying the metaphors, the therapist can focus on addressing the issues that were identified:

- Inability to eat around others/fear of judgement.
- Feeling alone and unsupported.
- Relationship with mother.
- Ineffective boundaries setting.
- Issues around communication.
- Feelings of worthlessness.

Let's take a look at some symbols that will help your client link these representations by using the Family Meal exercise. This will help shift your client's awareness to noticing symbols that exist but that they hadn't connected previously.

CLIENT EXERCISE: LINKING SYMBOLS FROM THE FAMILY MEAL EXERCISE

Now that you have completed the Family Meal exercise and drawing, let's dig a little deeper and practice using our curiosity to identify symbols and metaphors in the drawing. This will help you link symbols from the past to the present time to determine if any are still influencing the way you react to food today.

Objective: Practice identifying symbols and representations from childhood family experiences using the Family Meal exercise.

What you will need:

- Quiet calm room.
- Completed drawing of Family Meal Exercise.
- Completed journal responses from Family Meal Exercise.

1. Notice and observe your drawing. Notice the objects you chose to draw for this exercise.
2. In the chart below, list the objects that bring up any emotion for you. Then write the emotion next to the object. What do you feel this object represents for you?

Object	Emotion	Represents/Symbol
Example: *Empty Chairs*	*Sadness, loneliness, unloved*	*Reminder that I'm alone*
Microwaved Meals	*Sadness, loneliness, unloved*	*Mom, comfort, care*
My dog	*Uncared for, neglected, unworthy, not good enough*	*Myself*

3. Notice and observe your drawing. Notice the objects you chose to draw for this exercise.

4. In the chart below, list the objects that bring up any emotion for you. Then write the emotion next to the object. What do you feel this object represents for you?

See the completed example by Leah.

Linking Symbols Chart

Object	Emotion	Represents/Symbol

5. What was happening during this time? What other memories did this exercise elicit for you?

6. Describe the memories that gave rise to any significant emotions.

7. What are the emotions that go with this memory?

8. How do you feel these memories still affect you today?

9. How do you feel these memories affect your relationship and behaviors related to food?

10. What do you feel is still unresolved and needs to be addressed in therapy?

Therapist Tips:

- *Most clients struggle with identifying symbols/metaphors because it is an unconscious process, therefore, its best to complete these exercises together, talking it through with them. Most of the symbols are revealed while the client is sharing information with you and often clients will miss or have difficulty recognizing the metaphor. It is common for therapists to be able to identify the metaphor and help their client gain awareness by asking clarifying questions.*

Now that your client is starting to think about metaphors, let's delve a little deeper and learn how to decode meaning from specific foods your client may struggle with. When you can teach your client that foods have meaning, information, and messages from their soul, your client can better understand that food behaviors are not a moral issue.

Clients often feel that they're a terrible person for their behaviors, this adds to their guilt and so they eat to comfort themselves, and the guilt, shame, and disordered eating cycle continues. Decoding their food and hunger helps to show that they're not a bad person and that there are underlying issues that need to be addressed. This is key to stopping the cycle. This helps your client put their negative judgments aside and practice curiosity about their eating process.

Finding the Metaphors in Food

In Chapter 3, we identified physical hunger and emotional hunger. After learning how to differentiate between the two, we can check in with our bodies and locate a physical sensation that lets us know that we are physically hungry, and we honor our hunger. We practice mindful eating by noticing our physical fullness cues, taking another bite when needed and putting the fork down when we are satiated.

However, what if after checking in with body cues, we observe no sign of physical hunger and we still have a strong desire to eat? What should we do then? When we are not physically hungry, our food choices and how we interact with food can give us helpful information about what is happening to us emotionally. The desire to eat is out of an emotional need rather than a physical one. When this occurs, the food that your client chooses contains valuable information and can represent what they need emotionally need but do not yet have the awareness or language to describe.

Let's take a closer look at what this means using Tyra as an example.

Tyra is a single professional and came to see me after countless diets failed. "I can't stop eating at night. I've tried everything. I just can't seem to stop eating. I always eat a bowl of Cinnamon Toast Crunch Cereal with cold milk at night and I know I'm not hungry. If I don't eat it, I lie in bed and think about it the whole time. After I eat it, I fall asleep like a baby."

Tyra was given the worksheets that follow to complete between sessions so that she could practice decoding her food to uncover the meaning behind the obsession with the cereal. It was revealed, "Cinnamon Toast Crunch Cereal with cold milk reminds me of my Granny's homemade cinnamon bread. When I was a little girl, My Granny and I baked bread together. I realized that I've been so lonely lately. I miss having someone that has my back no matter what. Someone who loves me for me, and I can just be myself with. I guess it happens at night because I feel loneliest when its quiet and I'm all alone."

Tyra realized that the cereal represented the warmth and unconditional love that she received from her grandmother that she been longing for. After Tyra uncovered what she desired, she made an effort to leave work earlier and to create a more balanced schedule so that she would have time to cultivate closer connections with others. When the food metaphor is decoded, the food no longer possesses the same power it did. This is because it is no longer an unconscious process. Having the awareness allows Tyra to address the real issue. Ok. Now let's give it a try with your client!

CLIENT EXERCISE: DECODING EMOTIONAL HUNGER (PART 1)

Have you noticed that you tend to gravitate toward some types of foods and totally avoid others? What have you noticed about obsessing over one food and completely fearing another? When food brings up emotion for us in this way, it is an indication that the food is likely representing something else. This exercise helps us to practice finding the metaphor in our food.

Objective: To uncover the meaning behind the food

Directions: Complete the worksheet by answering each statement with a complete response under each example.

1. Identify a food that you tend to eat when not physically hungry or a food you tend to restrict or avoid. Using the same food, answer the questions using a complete sentence.
   Example: Pizza

2. What do you see when you look at that food? *Example, "When I look at pizza, I see yummy goodness. Nice warm and softness."*

3. What do you feel when you see this food? *Example: "When I see pizza, I feel nervous and anxious because I'm afraid I can't stop eating it."*

4. What is it about the food that you hate? *Example, "I hate that I can't stop wanting you."*

5. What is it about the food that you love? *Example, "I love you because when I eat you, I feel better."*

6. What does this food promise? *Example, "You promise me that I will be ok and comforted."*

7. What do you wish when you see this food? *Example, "I wish that I could eat pizza and not get affected by guilt afterwards.*

8. What do you trust or don't trust about this food? Example, *"I don't trust that you will be good for me."*

9. What does this food remind you of? Example, *"You remind me of late nights crying over my ex-boyfriend."*

10. How does this food help you? Example, *"You help me with the hard times, but you add stress because of how I treat myself afterwards."*

11. If you could say anything to this food, what would you say? Example, *"I'd say get out of my thoughts."*

12. How can you make peace with this food? Example, *"The way I can make peace is by listening to my body and eat when I am physically hungry so that I don't feel so bad."*

1. After completing the worksheet (Part 1), review your responses and underline words or phrases that have significance or bring up emotion. See example above.
2. Review all the underlined phrases or words and bring to mind a situation, time, or person that brings up similar emotional reactions from you.
3. Then identify the situation, time, or person by writing it down on the second half of the worksheet and complete the second half just as you did the first, but this time using the situation, time or place to complete the statements.

CLIENT EXERCISE: DECODING EMOTIONAL HUNGER (PART 2)

Directions: Identify a situation, time, or person that brought up similar feelings or emotions from Part 1 of the worksheet.

Complete Part 2 just as you did above in Part 1, however, this time using the situation, time, or person to complete the statements. Complete each question below each example in the box.

1. What situation, time, or person brings up a similar response in you? Example:
    Reminds me of my ex-boyfriend

2. What do you see when you look at the situation, time, or person? Example, *"When I look at my ex-boyfriend, I see a person that wasted my time."*

3. How do you feel when you think about the situation, time, or person? Example: *"I feel angry and upset with myself for not valuing myself."*

4. What do you hate about the situation, time, or person? Example, *"I hate that I couldn't get out of the bad cycle."*

5. What do you love about the situation, time, or person? Example, *"I don't love anything about it anymore."*

6. What was the promise from the situation, time, or person? Example, *"He promised that he was the only person that cared and only thing I deserved."*

7. What do you wish about the situation, time, or person? Example, *"I wish I would've seen my worth sooner."*

8. What do you trust or don't trust about the situation, time, or person? Example, *"I don't trust him at all."*

9. What does this situation, time or person remind you of? Example, *"Reminds me of how I knew I need to leave him but didn't."*

10. How did situation, time or person help you? Example, *"It helped me get away from my family."*

11. If you could say anything to this situation, time or person, what would you say? Example, *"I'd say I'm so glad I'm not in an abusive and controlling relationship anymore."*

12. How can you make peace with this situation, time or person? Example, *"Go to therapy and work on healing myself."*

After completing the second half of the worksheet, the meaning behind the food is revealed. If you are having difficulty with identifying the meaning, please follow up with your therapist and let him/her know where you need assistance.

What Happens after Your Client Uncovers the Metaphor?

When the meaning behind the food is uncovered, you can address the real issues with your client. You can also review the worksheet to identify any responses that you feel need to be explored further. The food will not have the same effect on your client once consciousness has been created. This exercise can be repeated any time your client is struggling with a specific food to uncover the metaphor. Most clients will find this exercise helpful. However, as you know, no one tool or exercise will help our clients master any skill. Therefore, it is important to have our clients practice skills using a variety of tools and exercises. This will help solidify their understanding.

Therapist Tips:

- *It's common for clients to have some difficulty doing this exercise on their own. This would be an exercise to do in session together.*
- *Once your client can identify the metaphor, your client will understand the value of these exercises and begin to look at food and their behaviors differently.*

Finding the Metaphors in Eating Disorder Behaviors

As mentioned earlier, your client will better understand how metaphors work in eating disorder recovery if they can apply it in various ways. We have reviewed how metaphors work with past situations and with specific foods. Now let's take a look at how metaphors can influence our client's unconscious mental processes. These are behaviors, thoughts, feelings, emotions, memories, perceptions, imaginations, or reasonings that your client may not be aware of that are influencing their choices and actions regarding food and body. These are behaviors that they tend to engage in that bring up intense emotions, usually indicating an emotional need that they may not know how to articulate or express in a conscious manner. The way in which your client engages in food holds valuable information on what might be going on in your client's life. When your client is able to decode the meaning behind the behaviors, it can take the power out of the behavior because the function of the behavior is no longer unconscious.

Let's look at a case example to illustrate this concept. *Marie is 21-year-old female, diagnosed with anorexia nervosa, had been in treatment for a few weeks, and had been noticeably engaging in consistent food rituals since her admission. Marie sat back and started to separate her food. She pushed her broccoli over to one corner, and carefully, with her fork, slowly moved each grain of rice over to the other corner of her plate. She separated her food consistently and it was obvious that she was uncomfortable with the various types of food on her plate touching. She pushed her cheese lasagna with her knife, carefully scraping the sauce, and pushing the sticky cheese to the other side.*

Marie then proceeded to eat. Slowly, her hands shaking, she would use her fork to play with her food, and she struggled with moving her fork towards her mouth. She took a deep breath and placed her for, back onto her plate, and repeated this process. At the end of the meal, Marie wasn't able to complete her minimum percentage of intake and was required to consume her prescribed supplemental drink.

Therapist:	*"How did dinner go?"*
Marie:	*"Not well, I had to take two Boosts. I just couldn't eat. My parents are coming this week and I know they'll be upset. They'll think I'm not making any progress".*
Therapist:	*"Tell me a little more about dinner. What was most challenging for you about dinner?"*
Marie:	*"I don't know. I guess all of it. The fact that I have to eat all that food. It's food that I normally don't like to eat. I don't like to eat food that's saucy".*
Therapist:	*"Okay, tell me more about what bothers you about saucy food?"*
Marie:	*"It's just so messy. It gets all over the place. It's runny and crosses into the other foods."*
Therapist:	*"Tell me more, what bothers you most about how saucy foods crosses over into your other foods? How much does that bother you from a scale of 1 to 10 with 10 being the worst?"*
Marie:	*"It's a 10. It's just gross. It contaminates all the other food. And I hate when my food touches. If I'm going to eat food like that, it needs to be in separate containers. I guess that's why I didn't eat. It was hard to eat my vegetables with sauce on it. And I don't like little grains of rice in food that shouldn't have rice in it."*
Therapist:	*"I see. You don't like when your food is touching, and you don't like when certain things are in something that shouldn't be?"*
Marie:	*"Yes, it all just feels so out of control. Do you know what I mean?"*
Therapist:	*"Yes, I would like to understand more. Could you tell me a little about what you feel has been out of control, and crossing over where it shouldn't be in your life?"*
Marie:	*"It's my whole life. I never really thought about it that way. But my whole life feels like that. I'm 21 now, and I still feel like everyone is in my business."*
Therapist:	*"Tell me more. Tell me more about how you feel like everyone is in your business?"*
Marie:	*"My parents. Mostly my dad. I don't get to say what I want, or what I feel. He tells me what I need to be doing. He tells me how to feel. He even tells me when I should go to the bathroom. He shouldn't be in my business!"*
Therapist:	*"How much does it bother you that Dad is in your business and you don't get to say or do what you want, from a scale of 1 to 10 with a 10 being the worst?"*
Marie:	*"It's a 10. I feel like I can't breathe and I'm starting to feel anxious just thinking about them coming this weekend."*
Therapist:	*"Okay, so you feel you don't have much control and or say about things especially with your dad? And you feel like he crosses your boundaries and is in your business when you don't want him to be, is this correct?"*
Marie:	*"Yes, I've given up on talking to him about it because we only end up fighting and his anger can be scary. I stopped telling him how I feel when I was like a teen."*
Therapist:	*"Would you say that saucy food would be like Dad, where he oozes and crosses into other foods?"*
Marie:	*"Exactly! I never saw it that way before".*
Therapist	*"Now when you think about your food touching, how much does that bother you now from a scale of 1 to 10?"*
Marie:	*"It still bothers me, but it bothers me less, maybe about a 4. It just doesn't feel as emotional now."*

As you can see, the process of Marie separating her food is a way to create space from her parents. The metaphor for Marie's process is that Marie needs to learn how to establish healthy boundaries with her parents, specifically her father. She feels overwhelmed by her relationship with her father and it is showing up in her food. Marie feels the need to control and separate her food to feel safe as though her food is not violating the space of the other foods on her plate.

This is a good starting point in helping Marie gain awareness about the underlying issues in the process of how she relates to food. Her process with food gives valuable information on what is going on in her unconscious and can be addressed once it is made conscious. This one example allows the therapist to understand that the following needs to be addressed and can be a good starting point in Marie's therapy.

- Relationship with parents, specifically father.
- Assertive communication, using her authentic voice, and establishing boundaries.

Finding the metaphor in food behaviors can be tricky at first, and it takes practice for both you and your client to eventually be able to see the metaphor clearly. It also takes practice as a clinician to ask helpful questions that will benefit your client. The most useful way to approach this is to always come from a curious, compassionate, kind standpoint. This helps model questioning so that your client will eventually be able to apply it for themselves and keeps their judgements from getting in their way of exploring their unconscious processes with food.

Now that we've looked at an example, let's explore process metaphors with our clients. A common struggle for our clients is with food rules, since most food rules are part of the eating disorder voice. You will learn more about these thoughts in the next chapter. However, if we attempt to decode food rules and to find the metaphor in the rule, we can begin to help our clients address the real issues rather than getting lost in the rule.

Food Rules: Process Metaphors

How often do we hear people say things like, "I am not really eating carbs these days" or "I don't eat past 7pm?" While these statements appear benign and are heard in everyday conversations, for people who struggle with eating difficulties, statements like these become rules that are lived by and if not followed brings up uncomfortable feelings like anxiety, shame, and guilt.

Food rules are loaded with information about what may be happening in our lives and what we would like to change. Decoding and finding the metaphor behind the food rule gives us information on why the rule exists. The function of all food rules is to create a sense of structure, safety, control, or predictability in what feels like a chaotic, ambiguous existence. These rules, if followed, promise less anxiety about our vulnerability in our environment, situations, and the people around us. Understanding the metaphor behind food rules allows insight about underlying issues that need to be addressed. When the issues are worked through, there is no need for the food rule to exist.

Note: sometimes food rules were created months or even years ago and the reason they had first developed may not even exist anymore, yet the rule still exists because the issues were never resolved. Therefore, the individual may have more difficulty with deciphering the metaphor in their current circumstance and may believe that the issue really is just about food.

CLIENT WORKSHEET: FOOD RULES

Those who struggle with food often have rigid rules around eating. But did you know that most of these food rules aren't about food? They're usually a metaphor for something else. A metaphor is a symbol that has a meaning different than what it appears to be. For example, the rule "I don't eat sugar" could be interpreted as a metaphor for "not being worthy of love (something sweet)."

Let's look at some common food rules and see if you can figure out the metaphor. Keep in mind that there are no right or wrong answers. Use your own life as a reference to practice finding the metaphor. For example, if you have never used the exact food rule indicated on the worksheet, imagine what could be happening or what you could be feeling that would lead you to using that food rule.

Directions: Review the common food rules below that have been shared by real people struggling with eating. Practice decoding what you think each food rule could represent.

Example:

Food Rule: "I have to eat with a small plate and short glass."
Metaphor: *There is way too much going on in my life right now and I need to keep things small so they're manageable.*

What do you think each food rule could represent? Answer below.

1. "I have to eat all meals before 7pm."

Metaphor:

2. "I only eat after working out."

Metaphor:

3. "I don't let myself get too hungry."

Metaphor:

4. "I avoid foods that have more than five ingredients."

Metaphor:

5. "The foods on my plate shouldn't touch each other."

Metaphor:

Metaphors behind the food rules are unique to each individual. However, the key below is an example of what to pay attention to so that you can explore with curiosity about your personal experience and finding the metaphor in the food process. Please note that issues with eating are complex, therefore there are various meanings. These are some examples of what each rule can mean.

Answer Key:
"I have to eat with a small plate and short glass."
Pay attention to "small and short", hinting there may be something that's happening in your life that may be big, overwhelming or unmanageable. The question then is, "What is happening in my life that I feel I need things to be smaller?"

"I have to eat all meals before 7pm."
Pay attention to "before 7pm." Hinting that there needs to be some sort of structure for the day. A question to ask, "What am I needing structure or control for? Does something feel chaotic, unstructured, or out of control? What happens if I don't eat before 7pm?"

"I only eat after working out."
Pay attention to only allowing yourself to "eat after working out." Hinting that you have to do something in order to earn food. Question to ask might be "What am I feeling I need to earn right now? What am I feeling undeserving about right now? What do I feel I need to make up for right now?"

"Don't let yourself get too hungry."
Pay attention to the words "get too hungry" What does hunger mean? What does hunger feel like and what happens when you get too hungry? These are some hints that can help you decode the rule. However, it is important to note that this food rule is a challenging one. For people who struggle with restricting food, this may be more of a reminder to make sure they eat (therefore, it is important that they are honoring their hunger cues). For someone who eats for comfort, this rule can help them feel safe by consistently eating and avoiding the sensations of feeling "too hungry." The question then is, "What has been feeling unsafe lately? Or what does the physical hunger sensations bring up for me? What am I afraid of that will get out of control?"

"Avoid foods that have more than five ingredients."
Pay attention to the words "avoid" and "more than" These are some hint words that lead you to ask, "What feels overwhelming? or What are you wanting or needing to keep simple? Or maybe what in your life feels complicated and you're needing to avoid?"

"The foods on my plate shouldn't touch the other."
Pay attention to the words "shouldn't touch the other." These words are hints and can lead you to ask, "what in my life do I feel like shouldn't touch the other? Or where do I feel like my boundaries have been violated? Or what happens and what do I feel if the food does touch the other?"

Again, these are just examples of questions that can help start your curiosity to both learn and find more meaning in what the food rules represent below the surface. With practice the meaning kind and compassionate towards yourself while learning.

Therapist Tip:

- *If your client gets stuck on a metaphor, ask them to tell you more about the rule. Pay attention to the way your client enunciates certain words and notice any changes in their tone as they speak. This will give you a hint about where you can ask questions for more clarity.*

CLIENT EXERCISE: DECODING YOUR FOOD RULES (PART A)

You likely have strict rules around food or eating. What are they? What do they mean? You might be surprised to learn that the meaning goes a lot deeper than what's on your plate. Let's explore them now.

Objective: To learn and gain insight about the function of food rules and the meaning behind them.

What you will need:

- Quiet room.
- Decoding Food Rules Exercise.

Directions: In the following exercise, complete the worksheet by identifying any food rules you have followed. Use the previous exercise as an example.

1. Think of a food rule that you have been following. Using the space under the bold wording "Food Rule" write down your food rule.
2. What do you think the food rule represents? Using the earlier exercise and key, practice decoding what you think the metaphor behind the food rule is and complete the next line using the space given.
3. Continue to identify food rules and do the same until all food rules are listed. Use more space if needed.
4. Then complete the questions found on Worksheet Part B.

---

1. Food Rule:

Metaphor:

What needs to be addressed:

2. Food Rule:

Metaphor:

What needs to be addressed:

3. Food Rule:

Metaphor:

What needs to be addressed:

4. Food Rule:

Metaphor:

What needs to be addressed:

5. Food Rule:

Metaphor:

What needs to be addressed:

CLIENT WORKSHEET: DECODING FOOD RULES (PART B)

Complete the following questions related to the previous exercise.

1. What did you notice about the process in which you completed this exercise?

2. Were you able to find the metaphor?

3. What did you notice about your emotions while completing this exercise?

4. Which food rules were most difficult/ most straightforward?

5. What insights did you learn about your food rules and what does it mean for you?

6. What are some insights that require more exploration and may need to be addressed?

7. How can you go about working on the real issue?

Therapist Tip:

- *Go over the completed worksheets with your client to get more clarity if needed. Both you and your client will be able to identify issues to work on.*

Now that we have learned the basics of how to decode and uncover food and food behavior metaphors, we will practice decoding metaphors in the following chapters, while merging in the other foundational skills. This will become more familiar for your client and will help make the function of the eating disorder easier to recognize. Let's take a look at the next chapter, where you will learn how your client's noisy thoughts affects their daily functioning. Foundational skill *#3 Quieting Negative Thoughts* is vital for helping your client through the next steps when uncovering the function for food and food behaviors.

Bibliography

Casasanto, D. & Gijssels, T. (2015). What makes a metaphor an embodied metaphor? *Linguistics Vanguard*, *1*(1), 327–337. https://doi.org/10.1515/lingvan-2014-1015.

Landau, M. J. (2018). Using Metaphor to Find Meaning in Life. *Review of General Psychology: Journal of Division, of the American Psychological Association*, *22*(1), 62–72. https://doi.org/10.1037/gpr0000105.

Malkomsen, A. et al. (2021). Digging down or scratching the surface: how patients use metaphors to describe their experiences of psychotherapy. *BMC Psychiatry*, *21*(1), 533. https://doi.org/10.1186/s12888-021-03551-1.

Rucińska, Z., & Fondelli, T. (2022). Enacting Metaphors in Systemic Collaborative Therapy. *Frontiers in Psychology*, *13*, 867235. https://doi.org/10.3389/fpsyg.2022.867235.

Thompson-Brenner, H. (2014). Discussion of "Eating disorders and attachment: a contemporary psychodynamic perspective": does the attachment model of eating disorders indicate the need for psychodynamic treatment? *Psychodynamic Psychiatry*, *42*(2), 277–284. https://doi.org/10.1521/pdps.2014.42.2.277.

Part III

Teaching Self-Awareness and Self-Acceptance Skills for Recovery

Chapter 5

Foundational Skill #3
Quieting Negative Thoughts

Effectively dealing with negative thoughts is one of the most important skills that your client will need to learn to fully recover from their eating disorder. Your client's inability to manage these thoughts can be a significant indicator for relapse (Zarychta et al. 2014). Teaching your client effective ways to eventually quiet negative thoughts are essential from the start of treatment.

I've found that breaking down this skill into the following techniques is most effective:

- Noticing and observing thoughts.
- Tracking triggers.
- Tracking coping tools.
- Noticing negative thought patterns.
- Singling out the eating disorder voice.
- Identifying the function of the eating disorder voice.
- Neutralizing, countering, and replacing the eating disorder voice.

I've also found that going in the order shown above tends to be most helpful for clients, since each one builds on the lesson before it.

The strategies in this chapter have roots in *mindfulness*: the intentional and nonjudgmental awareness of one's present-moment experience, including thoughts, emotions, sensations, and context (Kiken & Shook 2014). Mindfulness can foster a more adaptive and self-compassionate stance, especially when stress or adversities leads your client to disordered eating. One of the applications of mindfulness is to attenuate or neutralize negative cognitions, such as the *inner critic* and the *eating disorder voice*, both of which are addressed in this chapter. By practicing mindfulness, your client can learn to observe these cognitions with curiosity and acceptance, rather than endorsing them or reacting to them.

Your client can also learn to refocus their attention to more constructive and affirming aspects of their experience, such as in their relationships and their passions. This can diminish the impact and salience of eating disorder behaviors and enhance their wellbeing and recovery.

The benefits of mindfulness are rarely immediate, however; it's a practice that yields results over time. For this reason, at first, your client may feel discouraged, call the strategies ineffective, or want to give up. To help them stick to it, have your client practice the skills in this chapter anyway. Have them use the tracking worksheets or journal daily about what techniques helped them and what techniques did not.

When your client is able to articulate specific challenges, it is then easier for you to assist in refining exercises so they will be effective for your client. When your client knows that you will follow up and hold them accountable, they will be more cognizant while actually practicing a strategy knowing that they will be asked to reflect back on it.

Finally, it's important that your client practices all of these skills without judgment. This is a core tenant of mindfulness that encourages awareness and helps your client gain more insight about themselves. It helps develop the consciousness needed for full eating disorder recovery.

In this chapter, we will use the case vignette of Rachel to demonstrate how she built up her mindfulness skills through working with her therapist and completing various worksheets.

DOI: 10.4324/9781032651408-9

Case Vignette: Rachel

Rachel is a 29-year-old single female that sought help for her binge eating and restricting cycle. This is Rachel's fourth visit to her individual therapist.

Rachel: *"I've missed a lot of days at work. I just dread it so much. I feel really guilty about it and find myself eating. I feel terrible afterwards. I feel horrible about my body. I'm getting bigger and bigger. I know I shouldn't worry about my weight, but I feel so uncomfortable. My clothes are fitting tighter."*

Therapist: *"Okay, tell me about the worst day this week, what happened?"*

Rachel: *"I feel like all the other days were leading up to yesterday. I was worried about a meeting. I think my supervisor already doesn't like me. I don't feel confident. Everything feels overwhelming. I just can't handle what's expected of me and I don't feel like I'm doing a good job."*

Therapist: *"Tell me about your thoughts when you first got out of bed."*

Rachel: *"My thoughts were, it's too much, everyone thinks you're incompetent, you can't handle what they're giving you, you're an idiot, you have no clue what you're doing. You should just go back to bed."*

Therapist: *"Sounds like your negative thoughts were intense."*

Rachel: *"Yes, it was so mean, I just wanted to go back to bed and shut it all out. When I get like that, it's hard for me to move on with the rest of my day. I just want to shut down. I felt like I was going to have a panic attack, then I called out from work, and the worst part, I stayed home and binged all day. And then of course the thoughts got worse. That was basically my week."*

Let's go through the techniques one by one, using Rachel as an example.

Noticing and Observing Thoughts

In Rachel's case, her disordered eating behaviors can be attributed to a mean unabating negative voice that doesn't cease. She uses binge eating to cope with her intrusive negative thought processes (Verplanken & Tangelder 2011). Learning essential mindfulness tools will help Rachel successfully silence these thoughts.

This appears straightforward, right? Well, the tricky part here is that your client's negative thoughts have been an integral part of how your client thinks. Therefore, often your client doesn't know that they're experiencing negative thoughts, much less that their negative thoughts are directly connected to their maladaptive coping style.

This is why teaching your client mindfulness, being aware of and focusing on the present moment, accepting their feelings, thoughts, and bodily sensations without judgment is a crucial part of their recovery process. Helping your client build awareness of their negative thoughts by tracking them is the first step and this helps your clients see how their thoughts are connected to their emotions leading to unhelpful behaviors (Jenkins & O'Connor 2012).

When clients first start out with these exercises, they easily become overwhelmed because their minds are cluttered with noisy negative thoughts (Palmieri et al. 2021). Their eating behaviors help them to disconnect from their thoughts so it may be difficult for them to track them at the start of therapy. They often feel discouraged and may be avoidant of mindfulness exercises. Remember, eating problems are about checking out of their reality, so your client will be reluctant to connect to what's really bothering them. A helpful way to get your client started with mindfulness is to have them practice journaling daily. These daily journals can be used in your sessions to recall events that occurred during the week.

Therapist Tips:

- *Make sure your client completes the* Tracking Negative Thoughts Exercise *first, before completing* Tracking Triggers and Coping Tools.
- *You can go over this with your client or have your client complete the worksheet in between sessions to track their negative thoughts.*

Review Rachel's completed form before doing the worksheet with your client. It will help you to answer any questions your client might have about completing the forms.

RACHEL'S WORKSHEET: TRACKING NEGATIVE THOUGHTS WITHOUT JUDGMENT

What is my negative thought?	What am I imagining?	What am I noticing in my body?	What am I feeling?	What do I want to do?
Everyone thinks I'm incompetent, I'm an Idiot	Supervisor doesn't like me	Can't breathe, feels like a panic attack	Shame, guilt, embarrassment	Binging on food

CLIENT WORKSHEET: TRACKING NEGATIVE THOUGHTS WITHOUT JUDGMENT

All of us have negative thoughts from time to time. But sometimes these thoughts are so familiar to us that we don't see them as setting off a harmful chain reaction. Let's identify some of your negative thoughts and the role they may be playing in your life.

Objective: To cultivate consciousness and build awareness around disturbing thoughts.
Directions: Complete the questions in each box. Remember not to judge your thoughts.

What is my negative thought?	What am I Imagining?	What am I noticing in my body?	What am I feeling?	What do I want to do?

Tracking Triggers

After your client has successfully completed the Tracking Negative Thoughts worksheet, get them to do the same for the Tracking Triggers and Coping Tools worksheet. Keep in mind that people who struggle with eating typically struggle more with identifying the situation that caused the negative thought, which then triggered the chain reaction that led to disordered eating. When you think about it and look at all the elements happening simultaneously, it does make sense: it is easy to get distracted and taken away from what initially triggered this response. This is exactly the function of disordered eating: detaching from the activating event. Therefore, it is usually more challenging for your client to identify the trigger (next worksheet) than to recognize their negative thoughts (previous worksheet). Negative thoughts are obvious and hard for your client to ignore, so inviting them to track those first is a more effective starting point.

You will know when your client is ready for the next exercise. Often, your client will tell you something like, "Okay, so how do I get rid of the negative thoughts? Or "What can I do about them?" Then you can introduce the next worksheet.

For example, Rachel's real problem is feeling unsupported and overwhelmed in her job. She doesn't know how to communicate her needs to her employer and therefore judges herself as incompetent and other negative statements that leave her shutting down and avoiding the entire situation. Once the trigger has been identified, the therapist can address the real issue about "meeting with her supervisor." The therapist will continue to teach ways to quiet her negative voice while also utilizing the other foundational skills that are interrelated and needed in order to help Rachel learn to communicate with her supervisor. The other foundational skills that the therapist can work on with Rachel to help eliminate this trigger are foundational skills #6 *Understanding Myself in Relation to Others*, #8 *Using My Authentic Voice* and #9 *Changing My Story*.

Another benefit of this exercise is that it will give you and your client an idea of what kinds of activities your client thinks might help. Allow them to come up with their own solution and to practice it. However, it is not uncommon for your client to be unable to come up with an answer to "What can I do instead?" Rachel's answer is quite common.

If your client is unable to do come with an idea, encourage them to practice mindfulness exercises when they're not in distress. The following exercises will help your client learn to just notice without judgement. Also see foundation skill #7 *Coping with Emotional Triggers and Building Tolerance* practice tool ideas.

Review Rachel's completed worksheet before going over the next exercise with your client.

RACHEL'S WORKSHEET: TRACKING TRIGGERS AND COPING TOOLS

Trigger	Negative Thought	What am I imagining?	What am I noticing in my body?	What am I feeling?	What do I want to do?	What can I do instead?
Meeting with supervisor	Everyone thinks I'm incompetent, I'm an idiot.	Supervisor doesn't like me and wants to fire me.	Can't breathe, feel like a panic attack.	Shame, guilt.	Shut down, binge on food.	I have no idea. Nothing seems to work.

CLIENT WORKSHEET: TRACKING TRIGGERS AND COPING TOOLS

Your negative thoughts don't just come out of thin air. Most of the time, there's something—perhaps something subtle and beyond your awareness—that has triggered your negative thought. When you become aware of your triggers, you're in a better position to handle the negative thought. Let's look at some of your triggers.

Objective: To cultivate consciousness and track the origin of disturbing thoughts.
Directions: Complete the questions in each box. Remember not to judge your thoughts.

Trigger	Negative Thought	What am I imagining?	What am I noticing in my body?	What am I feeling?	What do I want to do?	What can I do instead?

Using Nature to Encourage Mindfulness

Spending time in nature can be a valuable and accessible way for your client to practice mindfulness (Djernis et al. 2023). Research has shown that being in natural settings can lower stress levels, improve mood, increase attention span, reduce negative cognitions, and promote well-being (Kiken & Shook 2014). Nature can also provide a rich and diverse source of stimuli for mindful awareness, such as sights, sounds, smells, and sensations (Karl & Fischer 2022). Environment can play a significant role for presence and increasing consciousness.

Help your client disconnect from distorted thinking patterns by asking them to observe something in nature. Afterward, have your client complete the worksheet. Later, this worksheet can be used to develop more realistic and effective coping tools customized for them. Over time, your client will not need to use the worksheet template, they will know exactly what is happening and they will be able to track their thoughts, feelings, behaviors effortlessly, a skill needed for full eating disorder recovery.

Therapist Tips:

- *Encourage your client to schedule this activity ahead of time to minimize disruptions. Remind them to be present and focused.*
- *Help your client make the connection that observing nature in a non-judgmental way is ultimately what they will need to be able to practice when noticing their thoughts. This helps them stay out of reactivity, by staying present and eventually utilizing other tools.*

CLIENT WORKSHEET: OBSERVE NATURE

Did you know that spending time in nature is one of the simplest ways to practice mindfulness? Research has also shown that it's very healing. In this exercise, you'll spend a short time in a natural setting observing something of your choosing.

Objective: Learn to notice without judgment.
Directions: Choose something in nature to observe. Spend 10 minutes simply observing, without judgment.

What did you choose to observe?

What did you notice about what you observed?

What did you notice about yourself during this process?

What did you notice about your thoughts?

What did you notice about your feelings?

What did you notice in your body?

The last part of the Noticing and Observing Negative thoughts process is trying something different and then recording the results. This is the Coping Tools Tracker. See Rachel's example below.

Tracking Coping Tools

While your client is continuing to practice mindfulness activities, such as observing nature (previous exercise), encourage them to track what is working. It may seem easy enough, but it is very likely that your client will have difficulties completing all prompts. However, this is a part of the process; with practice, awareness will eventually become effortless and natural for your client.

The key is finding something that works for them. If observing nature isn't proving to be an effective coping tool, encourage your client to try cross stitching, knitting, journaling, artwork, taking a walk—all of which can help with staying present.

Rachel learned that changing her environment is something that works for her. Being in nature helps shifts Rachel's attention to the present.

I practiced being mindful in nature. It was really hard. My negative voice was really loud. Going outside worked. It helped me get fresh air. It was hard to sit with my negative thoughts going in my head. Changing my environment and breathing.

CLIENT WORKSHEET: COPING TOOLS TRACKER

As you practice mindfulness—being in the present moment and observing, without judgment—it's important to keep track of what's working and what's not. After a while, you'll learn which mindfulness activity works best, so you have a go-to coping strategy when you need some grounding.

Objective: Increase awareness and identify effective coping skills.
Directions: Complete the questions in each box. Remember not to judge your thoughts.

What did I choose to do instead?	What did I notice?	What worked?	What didn't?	What do I need to practice?

Noticing Negative Thought Patterns

Incessant negative thoughts are commonly a characteristic of depression. Frequently, individuals struggling with food are also dealing with depression and anxiety. Eating disorder behaviors can be used to cope with and in turn worsen these symptoms. When individuals are dealing with this, their negative thoughts can be overwhelming. It is important to note that many suffering from perpetual negative beliefs deny feeling depressed, however they struggle with food. When clients learn that their negative thought patterns can alter their perception of reality, they will be able to recognize when they are falling into a negative thinking trap (Coelho et al. 2015).

RACHEL'S WORKSHEET: NEGATIVE THINKING PATTERNS

Cognitive Distortion	Definition	Give one example of how you've experienced this.	How does this thinking affect your eating behaviors?
Polarized Thinking (also known as All or Nothing Thinking, or Black and White Thinking)	*When you see the world in extreme and absolute terms, without any middle ground.*	*Yeah, like if I miss a day of work, I think I should just quit my job all together.*	*If I start eating, I might as well eat everything and start again tomorrow.*
Mental Filter	*When you focus on a single negative piece of information and excludes all the positive ones.*	*This happens a lot. I get praised for what I do at work and only focus on the one mistake.*	*Well, it's happening now. I dread going to work and feel so guilty about it, I've been binging to feel better.*
Mind Reading	*When you think that you know what another person is thinking.*	*Yikes, I guess this is why I don't want to meet with the supervisor. I think she hates me, but I really don't know.*	*I've been avoiding it and it's been making me sick, and I've just been eating.*
Fortune Telling	*When you make conclusions and predictions based on little to no evidence.*	*This goes with mind reading. I've been thinking she's going to fire me, but I don't have any evidence.*	*Same as above. I've been avoiding it and just eating food.*
Magnification (Catastrophizing) or Minimization	*When you exaggerate or minimize the meaning, importance, or likelihood of things.*	*Yeah, everything feels like it gets really bad for me, and I guess I always minimize the good things I do.*	*I feel anxious a lot and makes me worried about the outcome. I end up stress eating.*
Emotional Reasoning	*When you accept your emotions as fact.*	*I always think whatever I feel must be true.*	*Same I want to shut down, cause the feelings can be intense and then I eat a lot, and then I try to make up for it.*
Control Fallacies	*When you think that you either (1) have no control over your life and are a helpless victim of fate, or (2) are in complete control of yourself and your surroundings, giving you responsibility for the feelings of those around you.*	*I always feel like I have no control, and at the same time, I feel like I'm responsible for everyone. This is my work situation.*	*I didn't realize it, but I guess I feel I have no control when I binge and feel way more in control when I make up for it by not eating the next day.*

CLIENT WORKSHEET: NEGATIVE THINKING PATTERNS

No matter how hard we try, our mind sometimes gets stuck in a negative-thinking cycle. It happens to everyone. The good news is that by simply being aware of them, you can make the link between your thoughts and your behaviors—and eventually change the way you relate to food for the better. Let's look at seven negative thinking traps and how they keep you stuck.

Objective: to Recognize Negative Thinking Patterns and how it affects your Eating Behaviors
Directions: Complete the following worksheet and discuss with your therapist.

Cognitive Distortion	Definition	Give one example of how you've experienced this.	How does this thinking affect your eating behaviors?
Polarized Thinking (also known as All or Nothing Thinking, or Black and White Thinking)	*When you see the world in extreme and absolute terms, without any middle ground.*		
Mental Filter	*When you focus on a single negative piece of information and excludes all the positive ones.*		
Mind Reading	*When you think that you know what another person is thinking.*		
Fortune Telling	*When you make conclusions and predictions based on little to no evidence.*		
Magnification (Catastrophizing) or Minimization	*When you exaggerate or minimize the meaning, importance, or likelihood of things.*		
Emotional Reasoning	*When you accept your emotions as fact.*		
Control Fallacies	*When you think that you either (1) have no control over your life and are a helpless victim of fate, or (2) are in complete control of yourself and your surroundings, giving you responsibility for the feelings of those around you.*		

Singling Out the Eating Disorder Voice

While depression and anxiety can cause negative thoughts, worry, and rumination, the negative *eating disorder voice* is unique to people struggling with disordered eating (Pugh 2020). The loud critical voices, intrusive negative thoughts, negative self-talk and various critical voices altogether are known as the "eating disorder voice." These thoughts play a crucial role in your client maintaining their eating disorder (Scott et al. 2014). The eating disorder thoughts and eating disorder voice is defined as, "cognitions, inner verbalizations related to self-worth, eating behaviors, or weight and appearance" (Scott et al. 2014).

Without teaching your client about awareness of these thoughts and how to effectively deal with the constant blather, your client will likely feel defeated, and the eating difficulties will progressively worsen (Smith et al. 2019). If the eating disorder voice is not addressed and your client doesn't learn the skills to effectively quiet these thoughts and voices, relapse will likely occur (Aya et al. 2019).

Our clients have a tendency to struggle with these exercises at the start of treatment because they are not used to staying mindful and present. They often experience worry, rumination, and anxiety and therefore these voices and thoughts become functional for them. Often, clients that struggle with perfectionism or fear failure or rejection are hesitant about giving up this voice because they feel that it keeps them in line so that they don't mess up or gives them a sense of control—a perception that they can somehow prevent, embarrassment, rejection, humiliation, shame, or any other potential threat by fixing themselves before they're exposed by others.

The forms that the eating disorder voice may take are by no means exhaustive. The eating disorder voice shows up differently and coincides with unique situations. To help you have a better understanding, this list is an example of how the eating disorder voice appears to your clients (Forsén Mantilla et al. 2018).

- **As Friend, Seducer, or Mentor**
  - The tone is comforting, protective, and helpful.
  - The intensity is low, usually at onset of developing an eating disorder or when the eating disorder resurfaces after having been dormant for those that have had treatment. Could be an early sign of relapse.
  - It says, "If you lose weight, you'll be happier." or "You'll feel better after the bag of cookies" or "If you just throw it up, you won't feel so bad."
  - It causes your client to count calories, read food labels, ignore physical hunger and fullness cues. Ignores body's needs.

- **As Coach or Critic**
  - The tone is controlling and hostile. Viewed as helping with self-discipline and increasing morality.
  - The tone is medium, when the eating disorder progressively worsens and the voice becomes louder.
  - It says, "You need to lose a few more pounds, you can do it!", "You're weak for eating the bad food, "If you go over x calories, then get rid of the rest."
  - It causes your client to restrict food, compulsively exercise, judge foods as "good" and or "bad." Extreme guilt when overeating after restricting food.

- **As Punisher, abuser, or bully**:
  - The tone is punitive, relentless, and overwhelming. Undermines self-esteem and brings about self-doubt.
  - The intensity is high, voice is aggressive and belittling, constant, and loud.
  - It says, "You don't deserve food." "You are stupid", "You are a fat slob", "You are an idiot", "You are just taking up space", "You're worthless!"
  - It urges your client to severely restrict food, binge, and purge food. Overexercises, isolates from others, withdraws from social situations.

The eating disorder voice typically appears when individuals with eating problems are trying to avoid feeling or are dealing with something. The eating disorder voice acts as a way to distract them from the real problem, creating a different issue to focus on and helps them to avoid the issues that feel too overwhelming to address.

Rachel was able to complete the following worksheet, but only after having learned about the eating disorder voice and having practiced mindfulness. As you will see, Rachel recognized that the sneaky voice shows up when she feels unsure. This process has helped Rachel learn more about herself and what she may need.

Let's help your client gain awareness of their eating disorder voice and thoughts by having them complete the following worksheet and discovering what it's like for them. This will help you understand what they are struggling with and how intense the voices are for them. This is a great way to gauge where they are and to identify helpful interventions.

Therapist Tips:

- *Make sure your client has begun a regular mindfulness practice before introducing this exercise.*
- *With practice, your client eventually will be able to differentiate the subtleties of their eating disorder voice.*
- *Case examples will help your client recall their experience. It also gives your client an idea about how to complete the worksheets.*
- *Remember that it's common for clients to struggle with recalling these thoughts because they have worked hard to shut them out using maladaptive behaviors.*

RACHEL'S WORKSHEET: RECOGNIZING THE EATING DISORDER VOICE

What situation/event triggers this voice?	How do you view this voice? Intensity?	What does the voice say?	What ED behaviors do you engage in?
The sneaky voice comes up when I'm unsure about something.	*When it's quiet, I see the voice as sneaky. Sort of disguised as helpful (it's usually unnoticeable) so not that intense to start.*	*It is always second guessing me, like it always begins with "are you sure you want to eat that? Or are you sure you want to?"*	*Usually, I get more confused when I hear the voice, and then end up eating because I'm full of self-doubt and confused about everything.*
When I've been beating myself up or feel really bad about myself.	*It's like a critical boss kind of voice that's like "get it together." It can get intense.*	*Usually says things like, "get it together." "Start going to the gym and get rid of the food you ate."*	*I try to get it together. Sometimes, I may restrict for a few days, but other times, I may try going to the gym, other times, I just give up and eat because I don't think I can do it.*
When I've been using behaviors for a while and not doing anything productive and when I feel horrible about myself to the point of where I hate myself.	*The voice is so loud and mean. It is really abusive and aggressive. I feel so beat up and horrible, ashamed and don't want to be seen by anyone.*	*"You're a fucking idiot. You're disgusting, horrible, person that is worthless. No one likes you. They all talk behind your back. You don't deserve anything. You're gross. Look at your life. Just a loser."*	*I just cry and isolate. I shut down and hate the world. Then I say fuck it, and just eat, cause what's the point.*

CLIENT WORKSHEET: RECOGNIZING THE EATING DISORDER VOICE

What have you noticed about your eating disorder voice? How do you experience the eating disorder voice?

Complete the chart below. Can you identify the voice that shows up? Let's practice getting to know more about the voice and the behaviors that follow.

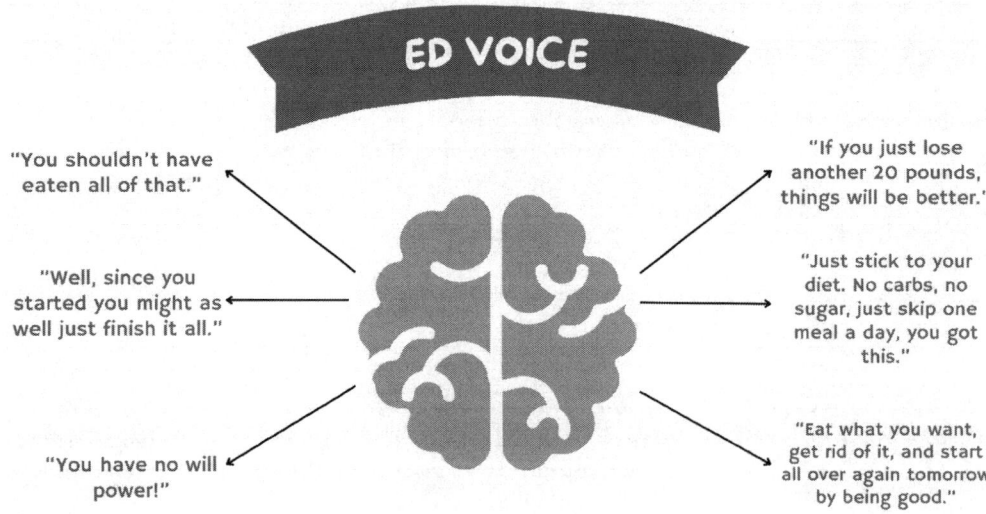

Figure 5.1 The Eating Disorder Voice

What situation/event triggers this voice?	How do you view this voice? Intensity?	What does the voice say?	What ED behaviors do you engage in?

Identifying the Function of the Eating Disorder Voice

So now that your client recognizes their eating disorder voice, then what? Many clients have had previous treatment and can recognize their eating disorder thoughts. However, these are the same people who have never learned what to do with them and therefore often relapse.

Let's first take a look at how the eating disorder voice can be functional so that you can work together to uncover what's happening on a deeper level. If your client tries to ignore the eating disorder voice altogether, often the voice will be more persistent. The eating disorder voice and thoughts can be reframed as a superpower and viewing it in this way helps your client to be less fearful of the thoughts. The eating disorder voice or thoughts is an indicator that something is wrong. When the voice or thought shows up, it is a prompt that your client may need to pause and take a deeper look at what is beneath the surface. The eating disorder voice can be seen as a layer of protection; that's its function. It's a hint to your client that they've been ignoring something important. Your client will need to pause and practice mindfulness so that they can uncover what they are really needing in that moment.

Therapist Tips:

- *When your client is done rating each statement on a Likert scale of 0 (not experiencing) to 7 (experiencing all waking hours), address the statements, prioritizing higher rated statements first, and work your way down to the lower rated statements. You will then be able to identify what your client struggles with most.*

Use this exercise in conjunction with exercises for foundational skill #4 Practicing Self-Compassion, Self-Acceptance, and Self-Care to further strengthen their foundational skills.

- *This exercise will also give you more information to better understand what to focus on with your client especially at the start of therapy.*
- *Often the unceasing voice can feel intense all the time for your client. When this occurs, look for themes for your starting point.*
- *Help your client identify coping skills that are realistic, doable, and enjoyable while working on challenging areas.*

First look at Rachel's example before exploring with your own client. This example has been modified to include therapist notes that further explain how to uncover what the function is behind the eating disorder voice.

RACHEL'S WORKSHEET: FINDING THE FUNCTION IN EATING DISORDER VOICE

1. **Promise (of reduced pain):** Example: *"If I'm thinner/lose weight, then <u>"I'll be happier."</u>*

   Rating: *7*

   (Therapist Note: Address dissatisfaction in her life, foundational skill *#9 Changing My Story.*)

2. **Consolation:** Example: *"I may not be doing so well <u>at work or in my relationships</u> but at least I'm thin."*

   Rating: *7*

   (Therapist Note: Address interpersonal challenges, foundational skill *#6 Understanding Myself in Relation to Others.*)

3. **Validation:** Example: *"I'm doing really well in controlling my food, so <u>I try to not let everything else bother me</u>...shouldn't bother me."*

   Rating: *7*

   (Therapist Note: Identify what she is avoiding foundational skill *#7 Coping with Emotional Triggers and Building Resilience.*)

4. **Threats:** Example: *"If I don't keep my eating under control, then <u>everything feels worse and out of control.</u>*

   Rating: *7*

   (Therapist Note: Address what currently feels out of control other than eating, foundational skill *#7 Coping with Emotional Triggers and Building Resilience.*)

5. **Cautious:** Example *<u>"Talking to my supervisor triggers my anger</u> and is dangerous, I'm going to have to be really careful about what I eat."*

   Rating: *7*

   (Therapist Note: Address foundational skill *#6 Understanding Myself in Relation to Others* and foundational skill *#7 Coping with Emotional Triggers and Building Resilience.*)

6. **Compensatory:** Example: *"I'm worried that <u>the stress and people at work</u> is too much, I need to get rid of it somehow."*

   Rating: *7*

(Therapist Note: Address foundational skill *#7 Coping with Emotional Triggers and Building Resilience* and foundational skill *#6 Understanding Myself in Relation to Others.*)

7. **Self-abuse**: Example: *"I'm so <u>hopeless, and a failure,</u> I have no self-control nor discipline.*

   Rating: <u>7</u>

   (Therapist Note: Address self-perception, foundational skill *#4 Practicing Self-Compassion, Self-Acceptance, and Self-Care.*)

8. **Self-punishment**: Example: *"Because I failed at <u>not going to work, I want to eat everything and just beat myself up all day,</u> I don't deserve to eat or partake in anything pleasurable."*

   Rating: <u>7</u>

   (Therapist Note: Address: foundational skill *#1 Establishing a Mind-Body Connection,* foundational skill *#2 Uncovering the Meaning Behind Food and Eating,* foundational skill *#3 Quieting Negative Thoughts,* and foundational skill *#7 Coping with Emotional Triggers and Building Resilience.*)

9. **Self-criticism**: Example: *"I'm such failure, I try so hard at <u>everything I do</u> but I'm just not the type of person I want to be."*

   Rating: <u>7</u>

   (Therapist Note: Address self-perception, foundational skill *#4 Practicing Self-Compassion, Self-Acceptance, and Self-Care* and foundational skill *#9 Changing My Story.*)

10. **Comparisons**: Example: *"Look at her, she's the perfect body type and I wish I <u>was more put together</u> just like her."*

    Rating: <u>7</u>

    (Therapist Note: Address self-perception, foundational skill *#4 Practicing Self-Compassion, Self-Acceptance, and Self-Care.*)

11. **Reinterpretations**: Example: *"When someone tells me I look <u>like I know what I'm doing,</u> what they're really saying is <u>they know I have no idea what I'm doing.</u>*

    Rating: <u>7</u>

    (Therapist Note: Address self-perception foundational skill *#4 Practicing Self-Compassion, Self-Acceptance, and Self-Care.*)

12. **Sensory misperceptions**: Example: *"Look at my <u>stomach</u>", makes me feel <u>like a failure.</u>*

    Rating: <u>7</u>

    (Therapist Note: Address body image, foundational skill *#5 Exploring Body Neutrality and Acceptance.*)

13. **Denial**: Example: *"My eating disorder isn't in control. I just need to <u>not shut down."</u>*

    Rating: <u>7 this is the hardest for me.</u>

    (Therapist Note: Address tolerating emotional distress, foundational skill *#7 Coping with Emotional Triggers and Building Resilience.*)

14. **Fear**: Example: *"If I let go of my eating disorder, I fear <u>I have no outlet."</u>*

    Rating: <u>7</u>

    (Therapist Note: Address emotional distress tolerance, foundational skill *#7 Coping with Emotional Triggers and Building Resilience.*)

15. **Judgments**: Example: *"If I don't look a certain way, people will think I'm <u>incompetent."</u>*

    Rating: <u>7</u>

    (Therapist Note: Address self-perception foundational skill *#4 Practicing Self-Compassion, Self-Acceptance, and Self-Care.*)

This worksheet exercise may take two sessions to complete. It is important to go over the completed worksheet with your client so that you can ask clarifying questions to better understand their unique experience. Once the function is revealed, you can then work on the underlying issues in subsequent sessions.

Have your client complete the worksheet below. They may have challenges with answering the questions, therefore, consider going over the case example with your client first so that it can help stimulate the necessary information.

CLIENT WORKSHEET: FINDING THE FUNCTION IN EATING DISORDER VOICE

Complete each statement with a word or a phrase that you've noticed in your negative self-talk, or your eating disorder voice. Then rate each statement on a scale of 0 to 7, where 0 means no experiencing of it and 7 means experiencing it at all waking hours.

Promise (of reduced pain): Example: *"If I'm thinner/lose weight, then* _____
_____ *"*

    Rating: _____

Consolation: Example: *"I may not be doing so well in*_____
but at least I'm thin."

    Rating: _____

Validation: Example: *"I'm doing really well in controlling my food, so* _____
_____*shouldn't bother me."*

    Rating: _____

Threats: Example: *"If I don't keep my eating under control, then* _____*.*

    Rating: _____

Cautious: Example *"*_____*(situation) is dangerous, I'm going to have to be really careful about*
what I eat."

    Rating: _____

Compensatory: Example: *"I'm worried that* _____ *(something other than food) is too much,*
I need to get rid of it somehow."

    Rating: _____

Self-abuse: Example: *"I'm so*_____*, I have no self-control nor discipline.*

    Rating: _____

Self-punishment: Example: *"Because I failed at* _____*, I don't deserve to eat or partake in any-*
thing pleasurable."

    Rating: _____

Self-criticism: Example: *"I'm such failure, I try so hard at* _____ *but I'm just not the type of*
person I want to be."

    Rating: _____

Comparisons: Example: *"Look at her, she's the perfect body type and I wish I had* _____ *just*
like her."

    Rating: _____

Reinterpretations: Example: *"When someone tells me I look _____, what they're really saying is _____."*

Rating: _____

Sensory misperceptions: Example: *"Look at my _____ (body part), makes me feel _____."*

Rating: _____

Denial: Example: *"My ED isn't in control. I just need to_____."*

Rating: _____

Fear: Example: *"If I let go of my ED, I fear_____."*

Rating: _____

Judgments: Example: *"If I don't look a certain way, people will think I'm_____."*

Rating: _____

Therapist Tip:

- *Refer to foundational skill #7 Coping with Emotional Triggers and Building Resilience for additional ideas on coping while dealing with underlying issues.*

Neutralizing, Countering, and Replacing the Eating Disorder Voice

We've explored some of what the eating disorder voice is about. Your client will still be quite distracted by the eating disorder voice, particularly if the voice is obtrusive. While your client is working in therapy to address the underlying issues, they will still have to learn ways to deal with the voice while these matters are being worked through.

First, remember an eating disorder thought is a prompt for your client to check in with themselves. Often, it means there's something bothering them and eating disorder thoughts surface to cope by detaching from their reality. Commonly, individuals will re-encounter eating disorder thoughts after having learned to quiet the voice. This leads to feelings of vulnerability fearing that urges to use behaviors will re-emerge. However, frequently, the eating disorder thoughts resurface because there is something the individual is avoiding. Taking a break and recentering often helps clients to reconnect to their self-care needs. This quality time helps them to realize what they've been dismissing.

Teaching this technique involves three exercises—Neutralizing Thoughts, Countering Thoughts, and Child-Self Imagery—with the worksheet Neutralizing, Countering, and Replacing the Eating Disorder Voice. It's advisable to have your client practice all three exercises before completing the worksheet.

Neutralizing the Eating Disorder Voice

When clients try to challenge negative thoughts when just starting out, the eating disorder voice argues louder and more aggressively. Therefore, neutralizing thoughts is a good place to start.

Have your client practice this exercise when noticing eating disorder voices or negative thoughts. Ask them to record results in the Coping Tools Tracker. There is no perfect way to do this and often your client will judge their performance. Remind them to be open and curious and not judgmental. Also, your client may not notice the effectiveness of the technique, because the absence of the negative thoughts is not as obvious.

Client Exercise: Neutralizing Eating Disorder Thoughts

Your eating disorder voice can be loud and persistent. When it is, practice this exercise so that it doesn't overwhelm you.

Objective: To neutralize the eating disorder voice, particularly when it is very strong, and return you to the present and a state of calm.

Directions:

1. When noticing eating disorder voice or thoughts, shift your attention to the present.
2. Ground by staying present and focusing on anything pleasant around you.
3. Look out the window, and repeat, *"the sky is blue"* or *"it's a sunny day"* or focus on something if indoors, such as the *"ceiling is white."*
4. Simply pay no attention to the eating disorder voice and continue to repeat in your mind whatever you chose to focus on, *"the grass is green"*, *"the walls are pink"* or the *"roses are red."*
5. Then imagine the eating disorder thought floating away on a cloud.
6. Continue this process whenever you notice the voice.

Here's what Rachel discovered using the neutralizing technique.

> *"The eating disorder voice was loud, and I just went on with my day and looked out the window and checked the sky and said out loud the sky is blue, checked the grass, the grass is green, and said it's a beautiful day. I don't feel great, but it's just a feeling and checking outside, lets me know it is ok. I can go on with my day and check back in later."*

In this example, Rachel is practicing skills in neutralizing her thoughts. She is not giving any attention to the eating disorder voice although she knows it's there. She will journal her thoughts and make a note of what she was doing so that she can check back later with her therapist to explore what the voice was about. In the meantime, her goal is to stay present, go on with her day, staying mindful. She is no longer reactive towards the voice and no longer strengthening the voice or thoughts by giving it any attention.

Countering the Eating Disorder Voice

For some, neutralizing techniques are highly effective. For others, the thoughts remain taxing and they will require other strategies to get rid of the voice. Countering thoughts will be helpful after practicing neutralizing techniques and they are more effective when used together. Therefore, when negative thoughts become louder and more aggressive your client will be able to move between the two techniques.

An effective way to counter thoughts is by fact checking what the negative voice is saying. For example, for people who tend to have restrictive tendencies, their negative voice is critical when it's time to eat. They often notice the eating disorder voice is triggered during mealtimes. Therefore, if the negative voice is saying, "You're always eating" the restrictive client will tend to have loud judgmental voices about food encouraging them to continue to restrict food. Your client can then do a fact check. They can check in with themselves by asking, "When did I eat last?" They can also fact check by asking themselves, "What sensations in my body are telling me that I'm physically hungry?" Countering the voice can then look like this, "Yes, the last time I ate was five hours ago and now I am hungry. My stomach is rumbling, and my hunger cue is at 3. It's time for dinner."

Here's what Rachel discovered while practicing ways to counter and replace the eating disorder voice.

> *"I practiced countering the eating disorder voice. The eating disorder voice said, I didn't deserve to eat, so I countered it by saying, "Yes, of course I do deserve to eat." And it got louder, and it said, "no you don't. You don't deserve anything! You binged last night so no you don't deserve to eat today!"*

Your client will need to learn to neutralize the eating disorder thoughts or voice before countering the thoughts because the eating disorder voice has a tendency to get worse. However, for some people, checking the facts is also helpful. For example, Rachel said:

"I noticed that when I countered my eating disorder thoughts, it was easier to do when I was able to check the facts. When my eating disorder voice got louder and more aggressive, I was able to challenge it by checking the facts. I responded to my eating disorder voice by saying, 'Well, today is a new day. Yes, I didn't listen to my body last night, but now it's breakfast and I do have a hunger cue, so I will practice honoring what my body needs.' It was so hard but it quieted the voice!"

For some, this technique is challenging because often individuals may be practicing assertions but don't actually believe what they are saying. In the next chapter dealing with self-perception, foundational skill #4 *Practicing Self-Compassion, Self-Acceptance, and Self-Care* will target the underlying reasons that cause the eating disorder voice.

Have your client practice the following exercise when noticing eating disorder voices or negative thoughts. Then ask them to record results in the Coping Tools Tracker.

CLIENT EXERCISE: COUNTERING EATING DISORDER THOUGHTS

Your eating disorder voice can be very critical and bossy. When it is, practice this exercise to quiet it down and lessen its power over you.

Objective: To counter the eating disorder voice—particularly when it is negative, critical, or judgmental—and return you to the present with less chatter.

Directions:

1. When noticing the eating disorder voice or thoughts, shift your attention to the present.
2. Ground by staying present and focusing on anything pleasant around you.
3. Look out the window, and repeat, *"the sky is blue"* or *"it's a sunny day"* or focus on something if indoors, such as the *"ceiling is white."*
4. Simply pay no attention to the eating disorder voice and continue to repeat in your mind whatever you chose to focus on, *"the grass is green", "the walls are pink"* or the *"roses are red."*
5. Counter the eating disorder thought by focusing on a fact: For example, your eating disorder voice might say, "You don't deserve to eat." Counter by "The last time I ate was at breakfast and its now noon, it is time for lunch, and I sense a hunger cue. I can honor my body's needs."

Replacing the Eating Disorder Voice

Commonly individuals struggle with having compassion for themselves. They feel unworthy and undeserving due to their self-perception. However, when they're able to connect to their childhood self, they do experience more compassion and less judgment. Therefore, this imagery exercise helps your client to connect to their younger self and counter the negative thoughts on behalf of their childhood self. This helps them to eventually be able to replace negative thoughts using their healthy voice. When your client is able to answer the questions in a compassionate way towards their younger self, they are ready to counter eating disorder thoughts with their younger self in mind.

When Rachel completed the Connecting to Your Child Self exercise, she had this to say:

"When I imagined my child self, I got so mad at the eating disorder voice. The eating disorder voice said, 'You're a loser, you don't deserve support.' I was so mad imagining the eating disorder voice scolding my little girl. I got so protective. I said, 'Yes, she does. She deserves support and she deserves my support too!' It was much easier for me to find my healthy voice."

Your client can also use the child imagery exercise if they are having difficulty with checking the facts. Your client will imagine the eating disorder talking to their childhood self, and they will counter and replace the eating disorder thoughts using their healthy voice keeping their childhood self in mind. As your client progresses in therapy, their healthy voice will increasingly become louder. This will be addressed in more detail in Chapter 9, foundational skill #8 *Using My Authentic Voice.*

CLIENT EXERCISE: CONNECTING TO YOUR CHILD SELF

If we aren't in the habit of checking in with ourselves, doing so can feel strange and even uncomfortable. But the truth is, you have an innate need for self-exploration. You already know how to do this. In this exercise, you'll check in with a younger version of yourself.

Objective: Connect to your child self and begin to replace negative thoughts from the ED voice with your healthy voice.

What you will need:

• Photograph of yourself at age three to five (preferably)

Directions: Take a moment to connect to photograph. Then answer the following questions.

1. What does this child need?
2. What does this child want to say?
3. What might this child be feeling?

RACHEL'S WORKSHEET: NEUTRALIZING, COUNTERING AND REPLACING EATING DISORDER VOICE

Eating Disorder Voice	Neutralizing Thought	Countering Thought	Replacing Thought using Healthy Voice
"You can't skip a day of exercise or you'll lose control and things will be out of control."	"The sky is blue and the sun is out." "I watch the eating disorder thoughts float away."	"I will move when my body wants to be active and rest when I am tired."	"I will check in with body and honor what my body needs."
"Since you already overate, you might as well eat it all."	"I imagine a heart and send eating disorder thoughts away."	"I don't have to eat it all now, since I am no longer hungry."	"I can live in the gray and don't have to be in black and white thinking. I can listen to my body and stop now."

CLIENT WORKSHEET: NEUTRALIZING, COUNTERING AND REPLACING THE EATING DISORDER VOICE

The eating disorder voice is deceptive! It can sound like a friend, a coach, a critic, or a bully. Either way, it is keeping you from having a healthy relationship with food. You can quiet the eating disorder voice by making a plan. In this exercise, you will map out the unhelpful things it says to you plus the helpful messages you can respond with.

Objective: To learn to recognize the negative messages from your eating disorder voice and identify ways to neutralize, counter, and replace it with a healthier message.
Directions:

1. Complete the worksheet by first identifying two eating disorder thoughts in the left column.
2. Then identify what you can do to neutralize, counter and replace the thoughts by recording your responses in each box.
3. Finally, identify which technique feels most comfortable for you and which technique feels most challenging.

Eating Disorder Voice/ Thought	Neutralizing Thought	Countering Thought	Replacing Thought using Healthy Voice

Next, let's continue to decrease negative thoughts and the eating disorder voice by connecting to Chapter 6, foundational skill #4 *Self-Compassion, Self-Acceptance, and Self-Care*. This will target negative thoughts from another angle that fuel problems with eating and body dissatisfaction.

Bibliography

Aya, V., Ulusoy, K., & Cardi, V. (2019). A systematic review of the "eating disorder voice" experience. *International Review of Psychiatry*, 31(4), 347–366. DOI: 10.1080/09540261.2019.1593112.

Bardone-Cone, A. M., Lin, S. L., & Butler, R. M. (2017). Perfectionism and Contingent Self-Worth in Relation to Disordered Eating and Anxiety. *Behavioral Therapy*, 48(3), 380–390. DOI: 10.1016/j.beth.2016.05.006.

Coelho, J. S., Ouellet-Courtois, C., Purdon, C., & Steiger, H. (2015). Susceptibility to cognitive distortions: the role of eating pathology. *Journal of Eating Disorders*, 3(31). https://doi.org/10.1186/s40337-015-0068-9.

Djernis, D., Lundsgaard, C. M., Rønn-Smidt, H., & Dahlgaard, J. (2023). Nature-Based Mindfulness: A Qualitative Study of the Experience of Support for Self-Regulation. *Healthcare (Basel, Switzerland)*, 11(6), 905. https://doi.org/10.3390/healthcare11060905.

Jenkins, P. E., & O'Connor, H. (2012). Discerning thoughts from feelings: the cognitive-affective division in eating disorders. *Eating Disorders*, 20(2), 144–158. DOI: 10.1080/10640266.2012.654058.

Karl, J. A., & Fischer, R. (2022). The Relationship Between Negative Affect, State Mindfulness, and the Role of Personality. *Mindfulness*, 13(11), 2729–2737. https://doi.org/10.1007/s12671-022-01989-2.

Kiken, L. G., & Shook, N. J. (2014). Does mindfulness attenuate thoughts emphasizing negativity, but not positivity?. *Journal of research in personality*, 53, 22–30. https://doi.org/10.1016/j.jrp.2014.08.002.

Mantilla, E. F., Clinton, D., & Birgegård, A. (2018). Insidious: The relationship patients have with their eating disorders and its impact on symptoms, duration of illness, and self-image. *Psychology and Psychotherapy: Theory, Research and Practice*, 91(3), 302–316. https://doi.org/10.1111/papt.12161.

Palmieri, S. et al. (2021). Repetitive Negative Thinking and Eating Disorders: A Meta-Analysis of the Role of Worry and Rumination. *Journal of Clinical Medicine*, 10, 2448. https://doi.org/ 10.3390/jcm10112448.

Pugh, M. (2020). Understanding "ED": A theoretical and empirical review of the internal eating disorder "voice". 10.53841/bpspsr.2020.1.65.12.

Scott, N., Hanstock, T. L. & Thornton, C. (2014). Dysfunctional self-talk associated with eating disorder severity and symptomatology. *Journal of Eating Disorders*, 2(14). https://doi.org/10.1186/2050-2974-2-14.

Smith, K. E., Mason, T. B., & Lavender, J. M. (2018). Rumination and eating disorder psychopathology: A meta-analysis. *Clinical psychology review, 61*, 9–23.

Smith, K. E., Mason, T. B., Anderson, N. L., & Lavender, J. M. (2019). Unpacking cognitive emotion regulation in eating disorder psychopathology: The differential relationships between rumination, thought suppression, and eating disorder symptoms among men and women. *Eating Behaviors, 32*, 95–100.

Verplanken, B., & Tangelder, Y. (2011). No body is perfect: The significance of habitual negative thinking about appearance for body dissatisfaction, eating disorder propensity, self-esteem and snacking, *Psychology & Health, 26*(6), 685–701. DOI: 10.1080/08870441003763246.

Zarychta, K., Luszczynska, A., & Scholz, U. (2014). The association between automatic thoughts about eating, the actual-ideal weight discrepancies, and eating disorders symptoms: a longitudinal study in late adolescence. *Eating and Weight Disorders, 19*(2), 199–207. DOI: 10.1007/s40519-014-0099-2.

Foundational Skill #4

Practicing Self-Compassion, Self-Acceptance, and Self-Care

Every therapist who has ever worked with eating disorders knows how challenging it is in helping their client change their negative self-perception. Negative thoughts and the eating disorder voice are strongly reinforced by your client's negative inner beliefs. People who struggle with eating and body image issues tend to view themselves as not enough, less than, a failure, incompetent, unlovable, unworthy, and undeserving (Williams & Levinson 2020). These are just some examples, but the list can be endless. Your client's feelings of inadequacy will undermine their recovery if not addressed.

In this chapter, we explore your client's self-perception, in order to help them better understand the origins and roots of their beliefs, how their perceptions affect their recovery, and how to heal towards self-acceptance. Your clients will complete practical exercises that help them to understand the origins of their negative self-perceptions (Meneguzzo et al. 2022), develop compassion in themselves, and learn how to turn the care they give to others on to themselves. I've found that the most effective way to teach clients these important skills is following this order:

- Assess how your clients view themselves.
- Unearth early maladaptive schemas (EMS).
- Teach self-compassion strategies.
- Teach self-care practices.

Assessing how Your Clients View Themselves

Let's take a look at Rachel's case example:

"My negative voice is harder to quiet down. The voice tells me, 'I'm just a failure, unworthy and unlovable' it's been loud since my boyfriend and I broke up. The thoughts all feel true. Why did we break up? I can't quiet the thoughts because it feels true."

In this example, Rachel is having trouble neutralizing, countering, and replacing her negative thoughts of "I am a failure", "I am unworthy", and "I am unlovable" because she is convinced these statements are real. The breakup with her partner substantiates her beliefs that she is a failure, unworthy, and unlovable—otherwise, why would her partner end the relationship?

Viewpoints such as these are typical with individuals who struggle with eating problems. This example shows that Rachel likely has negative core beliefs that are activated by emotionally distressing situations, known as early maladaptive schemas (EMS). It is helpful for your client to understand how early maladaptive schemas affect thoughts and self-perception and this will help them understand their origin (Joshua et al. 2023). This will also give them a better understanding of how these occurrences affect their urges to use maladaptive eating behaviors (Ansari et al. 2020).

Let's get started by learning how your client currently perceives themselves. The following exercise will help your client reflect on their self-perception, self-concept, and self-esteem. It's also a good starting point in exploring negative beliefs and potential obstacles in your client's treatment. This will also give you a better understanding about what your client needs and is helpful information in giving you a framework for the next skills.

DOI: 10.4324/9781032651408-10

Therapist Tip:

- *When doing this exercise following an emotional distressful event, your client's responses for negative inner core beliefs will be activated and will therefore be easier to identify.*

CLIENT EXERCISE: THREE PERSPECTIVES OF SELF, DRAWING

Sometimes it's easier to express ourselves in shapes rather than words, especially when the subject is ourself. Invite feelings of curiosity, freedom, creativity, and honesty as you draw.

Objective: Explore existing beliefs about your self-perception.
Directions: Complete each box by drawing an image that represents

- How you view yourself.
- How you think others view you.
- How you would like to be viewed by others.

After completing the drawing exercise, complete the Three Perspectives of Self Worksheet. Use Rachel's completed worksheet as a guide.

How I view myself	*How I think others view me*	*How I'd like to be viewed by myself and others*

RACHEL'S WORKSHEET: THREE PERSPECTIVES OF SELF, WORKSHEET

1. I see myself as: *It depends on the day. But mostly see myself as "not good enough."*
   And that I'm not as competent that I think I am. I'm fooling others but when they really see who I am, they leave me.
2. Others view me as: *I think others view me in two ways. There are the ones that believe in me and see me as competent, but when they get to know me, they realize they are wrong, and there are others that judge me right off the bat that "I'm not competent."*
3. I would like to be viewed as: *worthy, loveable, competent, enough and respectable.*
4. What makes you see yourself this was: *It just feels this way. I feel it in my body. I think it might be shame, like I was found out or something. When I'm rejected, I feel found out, like they saw the real me.*
5. What makes me think others view me this way: *It just feels that way. It's happened a few times. It's been a pattern. People are nice to me when they don't know me, but when they know me better, they leave.*
6. How does this perception of myself affect my relationship with food: *It usually makes me lose my appetite at first. I don't feel hungry, just sick to my stomach, and then later I can't stop eating, and just feel like a failure.*
7. How does this perception of myself affect my life, relationships, work, school: *It makes me want to isolate. I don't want to put myself out there. I fear judgment and rejection from other people.*
8. How does this perception of myself affect the way I think, feel, and my actions: *It makes me constantly judge myself. It makes me feel ashamed and it makes me want to isolate and not be seen by others. When I isolate, I usually eat to feel better.*

CLIENT WORKSHEET: THREE PERSPECTIVES OF SELF, WORKSHEET

After you have finished the Three Perspectives of Self drawing exercise, complete each sentence.

1. I see myself as…

2. Others view me as…

3. I would like to be viewed as…

4. What makes me see myself this way…

5. What makes me think others view me this way…

6. How does this perception of myself affect my relationship with food…

7. How does this perception of myself affect my life, relationships, work, school…

8. How does this perception of myself affect the way I think, feel, and my actions…

Unearthing Early Maladaptive Schemas (EMS)

In the previous example, Rachel holds negative core beliefs that are sparked by feelings of rejection from interpersonal situations. The underlined responses on her worksheet shows that Rachel's negative core beliefs—incompetence, unworthiness, being unlovable, defectiveness—are rooted in her experiences of perceived rejection and abandonment. These negative core beliefs have been developed from early maladaptive schemas (EMS) (Basile et al. 2019).

EMS were first identified by Jeffery Young. These are dysfunctional and pervasive emotional and cognitive patterns that were set in early childhood. They are the result of negative experiences with significant others, including core beliefs, emotions, physical sensations, and memories, that unconsciously lead to dysfunctional coping strategies preventing individuals from meeting their needs later in life (Gerges et al. 2022).

People who struggle with eating problems are characterized by their cognitive distortions and maladaptive schemas. These pervasive schemas, developed and adaptive in childhood and which function like "short cuts," relate to Rachel's early unmet emotional needs, consequently affecting and causing dysfunctional patterns in her current life (Legenbauer et al. 2018).

An important step is helping your client to understand their early maladaptive schemas. When your client understands the source of their negative inner beliefs, the connection to their childhood experiences, and how parallel negative experiences can trigger earlier reactive responses, this will ripple in three important ways:

- **The client can better identify current triggers.** They will be better at making distinctions and recognizing that their old dormant beliefs are separate but can be ignited by familiar negative patterns they experience in their current interactions.
- **The client can see the distinction between past behaviors and current emotions.** This awareness allows your client to identify and differentiate between reactions having to do with their past and current feelings that have been triggered.
- **The client can better self-regulate.** Awareness of EMS prevents emotional bombardment of combined past and current emotions and is therefore a tool your client can use to manage distressing situations.

Let's start by helping your client make connections and get a better understanding of early maladaptive schemas (EMS).

In our next exercise, your client will learn the origin of their EMS. Your client will develop consciousness about their negative beliefs, and then be able to recognize where their EMS stems from. Review Rachel's completed worksheet before inviting your client to complete it.

Therapist Tips:

- *This exercise is most effective when your client is actively experiencing intense negative thoughts, beliefs, emotions, or sensations.*
- *If you are a provider that is trained in eye movement desensitization reprocessing (EMDR), this would be an opportunity to target these negative cognitions. This will make the process of eliminating these negative core beliefs quicker. You can also always refer to an EMDR provider as well to target these negative core beliefs.*
- *This exercise can be repeated to target all negative beliefs.*

RACHEL'S WORKSHEET: ORIGIN OF NEGATIVE INNER CORE BELIEFS

Describe a current situation that brings up intense negative thoughts, beliefs, emotions, or sensations.

My boyfriend told me he wants to take a break. My negative thoughts are that I'm not lovable. I'm not good enough. I feel like anyone that gets to know me leaves me. This has been my pattern. I've never really had a long-term relationship. I feel really sad, rejected, betrayed, stupid for believing him. My heart hurts. I feel anxious. I have this lump in my throat and feel sick to my stomach.

What about this situation bothers you the most? What does this situation remind you of?

I can't believe this is really happening. And at the same time, it is. I guess what bothers me the most is I trusted him, and it took a long time for me to trust and open up to him. I feel really stupid. I feel like I should have known better. I feel betrayed.

I never really thought about this before now, but it's weird because it reminds me of my mom. It reminds me of the many times my mom lied to me. She would tell me to wait for her and she would leave. I'd wait for her, but she'd be gone and I was left. She would leave me at the mall or at a friend's house. I was never a priority.

What bothers you most about this situation? What does this say about you? (What is the negative thought that comes up about you?) For example (I am…) From a scale of 1–10 where 10 bothers you the most, identify the negative cognition that bothers you closest to a 10.

That's easy. The thing that bothers me the most is that I never mattered. It felt like I wasn't worth it or I didn't deserve to be taken care of or loved. I'm undeserving of love and care.

Using the negative cognition above, identify either the first time or the worst time you felt this way? What was the situation?

I've had so many times that I felt betrayed by my mother. I never felt I mattered. I listed an example above.

How old were you when this occurred? Who were the people involved?

This happened all through my childhood. I was probably five years old when she would always leave me and lie to me. I don't remember my mom being there. She would leave me with my grandmother a lot. I would cry to my grandmother. Or she would leave me at random places. I would just keep my feelings to myself, but I would feel sick like worried and with a stomach ache.

What was the worst thing about this situation? What was the negative cognition? (I am…)

The worst thing about it was that I had no one to tell. I had to hold it in and pretend I was ok when I really felt sick and worried and scared.

The scary negative cognition was "I am alone." That's still so scary for me.

What did you need or want to have happened?

I needed my mother to care about me. I needed her to take care of me and I needed her to follow through whenever she made promises. I needed her to do the things she said she would. I needed to be able to count on her.

As you can see in Rachel's responses, the breakup with her partner reactivated her negative core message of her unworthiness. Rachel's early maladaptive schema has to do with her childhood experience of feelings that her mother was unreliable. Rachel fears being alone, because being alone is confirmation that she is not deserving of love. Rachel's current negative thoughts and the intensity of her emotions feels analogous to her early childhood pattern. The unconscious affective memories from her past are compounded with her current feelings of rejection causing dysphoria.

CLIENT WORKSHEET: ORIGIN OF NEGATIVE CORE BELIEFS

Often we have negative core beliefs that operate outside of our awareness. They've been part of us for so long that we don't question them. The problem is, many negative core beliefs developed in childhood and no longer apply in adulthood. In this exercise, you'll reflect upon current difficult situations that have roots in your past and unearth how certain beliefs are negatively impacting you today.

Objective: Increase awareness of the origin of negative inner core beliefs.
Directions: Complete the worksheet below by answering the following questions. Remember not to judge any of your responses, and to complete all exercises with open curiosity.

Describe the current situation that brings up intense negative thoughts, beliefs, emotions or sensations.

What about this situation bothers you the most? What does this situation remind you of?

What does this situation say about you? What are the negative thoughts that comes up about you? For example ("I am…") On a scale of 1–10 where 10 bothers you the most, identify the negative belief that bothers you closest to a 10.

Using the negative cognition above, identify either the first time or the worst time you felt this way? What was the situation?

How old were you when this occurred? Who were the people involved?

What was the worst thing about this situation? What was the negative cognition? (I am…)

What did you need or want to have happened?

Now that your client is able to identify the origin of their negative core beliefs, what's the next step? Your clients can acknowledge that their early emotional needs were not met, however it is often challenging for them to show love, kindness, and tenderness towards themselves; as a result of their negative inner core beliefs they adhere to "I don't deserve it" (Yakın et al. 2019). Therefore, while they can pinpoint the origin for their maladaptive schema, they will still have trouble changing their self-view without first developing self-compassion (Kelly et al. 2013).

This is the second step in helping your clients change their negative self-perception.

Teaching Self-Compassion Strategies

Self-compassion as described by Kristin Neff comprises the ability "to respond to one's suffering by adopting, an attitude of caring kindness rather than judgment, viewing one's pain as common within humanity rather than isolating, and being mindful of one's inadequacies rather than ruminating on failures (Neff 2023).

People who struggle with eating issues have a tendency to judge their mistakes and suffering harshly. They often struggle to treat themselves with tenderness fearing that having self-compassion will reveal their flaws, acknowledge that they're weak, are emotionally vulnerable, or may have to deal with deeper hidden issues such as grief and anger (Gellaer et al. 2022). Therefore, it is known that people who have eating difficulties also tend to have low levels of self-compassion (Dias et al. 2020). Research shows that it's not just a deficit of self-compassion that hinders *eating disorder* recovery but also a fear of self-compassion (Kalika et al. 2022).

It is known that those struggling with disordered eating have perfectionistic tendencies. This aligns with their early maladaptive schema, themes such as failure, rejection, being unlovable, unworthy, or incompetent. This leads to erroneous thoughts that if they show kindness, understanding, tenderness, and love for their mistakes or for their imperfections, they are somehow unjustly letting themselves off the hook, or they fear that their perceived poor performance will be accepted as the norm, resulting in a lower personal standard (Fresnics et al. 2019). For them, the lower standard confirms their negative inner beliefs from their early maladaptive schema.

Many with eating difficulties also mistakenly believe that treating themselves with love and kindness will be viewed as narcissism. They may have close family members with toxic traits who have criticized them or judged them as selfish for having their own needs.

However, self-compassion is associated with positive mental health and has been shown as a required component for eating disorder prevention and recovery. Self-compassion is self-esteem and is unrelated to narcissism (Kelly et al. 2014).

Developing self-compassion is key in helping your clients quiet their negative voice and thoughts and work through outdated early maladaptive schemas. Studies have shown that people with higher levels of self-compassion experience lower levels of shame and have higher self-acceptance, which is a protective factor against body image distress (Braun et al. 2016). However, due to your clients' misconceptions, they will likely experience challenges when initially accessing compassion for themselves. Therefore, it is important to encourage your clients to practice daily exercises that support self-compassion, such as self-acceptance and self-care.

First, let's start by gauging your client's current level of self-compassion. Review Rachel's completed worksheet first, because it will give you some clues as to how your client might respond.

RACHEL'S WORKSHEET: SELF-COMPASSION ONLINE QUIZ

---

1. What was your self-compassion quiz score?

   Self-kindness: 1.00
   Self-judgment: 4.20
   Common humanity: 1.75
   Isolation: 4.50
   Mindfulness: 1.25
   Over-identification: 4.25
   Overall score: 1.51

2. What does this score tell you about your current level of self-compassion?

   I'm low in self-compassion.

3. What are your thoughts or feelings about the results?

   I'm not surprised at all.

4. What thoughts, feelings, behaviors did you notice while taking the quiz?

    I noticed I was getting down on myself and just wanted to just click on any response to get it over with.

5. How do you feel your level of self-compassion is related to how you view yourself?

    It's completely related. I have low self-compassion, and no patience for myself.

Rachel's responses and self-compassion quiz results help her to understand where her attitude is and how she treats herself in times of distress. This awareness lets her know that she has a tendency to be self-critical. While this may appear obvious to clinicians, people who struggle with low self-compassion have misconceptions that this is typical for others as well.

CLIENT WORKSHEET: SELF-COMPASSION ONLINE QUIZ

When you make a mistake or have difficulty with a task, how do you treat yourself? Do you tend to be harsh or empathetic? Let's find out where you stand on the self-compassion spectrum.

Objective: To get a baseline idea of where you are with practicing self-compassion.
Directions: Go to Dr Kristin Neff's website (https://self-compassion.org>self-compassion-test). Take the online Self-Compassion Quiz to determine your current score. This score gives you a general idea and a good starting point for further developing self-compassion.

After taking the quiz, answer the questions, below. Remember not to judge any of your responses, and to complete all exercises with open curiosity.

1. What was your Self-Compassion Quiz Score?

2. What does this score tell you about your current level of Self-Compassion?

3. What are your thoughts or feelings about the results?

4. What thoughts, feelings, behaviors did you notice while taking the quiz?

5. How do you feel your level of self-compassion is related to how you view yourself?

Now that you have an idea of your client's attitude towards self-compassion, we can move on to the next exercise. It is important to identify your clients' unique fears and judgments about developing self-compassion so let's take a look at the obstacles preventing your client from practicing it. These obstacles need to be addressed so that your client can work through any existing blocks. Let's examine how Rachel completed the worksheet before sharing it with your client.

RACHEL'S WORKSHEET: BARRIERS TO SELF-COMPASSION

---

1. What are some fears or negative beliefs you have about practicing self-compassion?

   I am feeling sorry for myself. It's like I'm telling everyone I'm weak.
   Also, people around me tell me to just "grow up" and stop acting like a baby.
   I don't want to be a victim. I was told, "stop acting like a victim."

2. Identify people (real, famous, or even characters in books or movies) that embody self-compassion.

   I have to be honest here. This was a really hard question. I felt judgmental with people.
   I feel less judgmental when I see this in animated films or with animals like dogs.
   I guess, I can see self-compassion in the Disney princesses, Belle from Beauty and the Beast, Cinderella and Mulan.

3. What qualities or traits did you observe to conclude that these people are self-compassionate?

   Belle didn't beat herself up and wasn't negative about her whole experience. She comforted herself when she was afraid, and she had compassion towards the beast.
   Cinderella was treated unkindly by her stepmother and stepsisters, and she made the best of it, and wasn't mean to herself.
   Mulan was a warrior. She honored herself and her experience.

4. Notice your fears and negative beliefs that you identified in box #1, what fears and negative beliefs that you have are observed in the people you have identified embodying self-compassion?

   It's funny because I only identified animated characters, and I don't see how my fears or negative beliefs show up in the characters at all.

5. What evidence do you have that your fears and negative beliefs about self-compassion are true?

   I only have my experiences that I shared in box #1, but I guess it could be untrue, because it might be just the people that I've surrounded myself with. I guess my mom doesn't have healthy self-compassion either.

As you can see, Rachel's judgments with self-compassion kept her from identifying real people that embody this characteristic. However, in exploring this, it helps Rachel think about and notice self-compassion in others. This creates consciousness for Rachel in reflecting on her own self-compassion.

CLIENT WORKSHEET: BARRIERS TO SELF-COMPASSION

If you find it difficult to be kind to yourself, you're not alone. However, self-compassion is available for all of us. Often there are obstacles—such as fears or judgment from the eating disorder voice—that get in the way of self-compassion. But like any obstacle, with awareness and skill you can overcome them.

Objective: To identify obstacles that can hinder self-compassion.

Directions: Answer the questions below. Remember not to judge any of your responses, and to complete all exercises with open curiosity.

1. What are some fears, or negative beliefs you have about practicing self-compassion?

2. Identify people (real, famous, or even characters in books or movies) that embody self-compassion.

3. What qualities or traits did you observe to conclude that these people are self-compassionate?

4. Notice the fears and negative beliefs that you listed in the question #1. Have you observed any of these same fears and negative beliefs in the people you identified in question #2?

5. What evidence do you have that your fears and negative beliefs about self-compassion are true?

Teaching Self-Care Practices

Self-compassion enables the emotion regulation necessary for using coping strategies such as acts of self-care when facing difficulties. Reciprocally, when these skills are practiced, self-nurturing and kindness is strengthened.

Those with early maladaptive schemas around themes of sensitivity to rejection and abandonment have more difficulty with self-care (Spirou et al. 2022). This is seen more frequently in people who struggle with disordered eating. As Rachel said:

> "*It's pretty simple, people who love you, care about you and want to take care of you. When my boyfriend lets me down by not following through on something I need, like food, or when he doesn't pick me up on time, I get so upset. I feel like I don't matter, or I easily lose my appetite because it's such a chore for him bring me food. I just don't want to eat anymore.*"

In this example, Rachel feels uncared for when her boyfriend doesn't follow through on the kind acts that he had agreed on. When her boyfriend reneges on a promise, it feels similar to the early maladaptive schema "I don't matter" revealed earlier when Rachel's mother failed to follow through on her promises. This pattern makes it more challenging for Rachel to want to do things for herself, because Rachel suffers from existing wounds from her unmet childhood emotional needs.

Rachel feels cared for when a loved one meets her emotional needs. However, when a favor is not fulfilled, it activates her negative belief pattern. How these patterns affect Rachel's interpersonal relationships will be addressed in more depth in Chapter 8, foundational skill #6 *Understanding Myself in Relation to Others*. In this chapter, the focus is on Rachel learning to treat herself the way she yearns to be treated by others where the obstacle is Rachel's negative belief: that she is only worthy if someone else is taking care of her.

"I am unworthy when people don't follow through. It doesn't help me feel better when I have to do it. I want my boyfriend to do it for me. I feel cared for and loved when he does it. Why should I have to do those things for myself. I want to feel like I matter and that I am worthy."

Rachel needs to practice caring for herself in the way she desires others to care for her. The dilemma here is that she has no desire to take care of herself. The beliefs are reinforced that she doesn't deserve to be taken care of which allows her to continue to feel bad about herself. She is stuck in a cycle, dependent on others for care, while negative thoughts surface congruent with the way she feels.

When Rachel can treat herself tenderly, then positive thoughts can follow. This is accomplished by practicing daily self-care activities which will in turn help to cultivate self-compassion and self-acceptance.

Practicing self-care activities to cultivate self-acceptance and strengthen self-compassion is important because it requires your client to practice skills using cognitive dissonance that can help create habits in forming new, and rewiring old, neural patterns (Ferreira et al. 2014).

For example, Rachel will experience discomfort practicing her new self-care activity because this behavior is inconsistent with her thought and belief of "I'm unworthy" resulting in cognitive dissonance. Due to this tension, Rachel's attitude and feelings will change so that her thoughts and her behaviors are consistent, thereby reducing her unease.

Over time, she will experience dissonance when speaking negatively towards herself and when she is treating herself in loving and caring ways which is what makes the time taken doing this activity important. When Rachel is consistent with these activities, repeating positive affirmations, self-acceptance and self-compassion will be more accessible.

So, let's introduce your client to a self-care activity. Have your client continue to choose self-care activities until they have noticed a positive change or until self-care activities have become a part of their daily routine.

CLIENT ACTIVITY: SELF-CARE FOR THIRTY DAYS

Are you ready for some TLC? Setting aside time to tend to your needs is vital to your whole health. For this activity, you make yourself a priority. This may be new and feel challenging, but with time you'll discover something transformative: The more time you spend meeting your needs, the more time you can show up authentically for others.

Directions: Choose a simple self-care activity that is enjoyable and realistic to do for 30 days. Here are some ideas.

- Applying a pleasant-scented lotion before bed.
- Brushing your hair daily.
- Taking a 30 minute mindful walk.
- Stretching daily.
- Gently washing your face daily.
- Taking a bubble bath.
- Morning meditation for 30 minutes.
- Relaxation breaks daily.
- Reading for fun.
- Walking in nature.
- Going for a daily swim.
- Yoga.
- Dance.

1. Do this for thirty days.
2. After each Self-Care activity, complete the Self-Care Observations worksheet to keep a journal log so that you can talk about this with your therapist.

CLIENT WORKSHEET: SELF-CARE OBSERVATIONS

---

1. What Self-Care activity did you choose?

2. How long did the self-care activity take?

3. What thoughts or feelings did you notice while engaging in self-care?

4. What would you like to add or change in your next self-care practice?

It is important to check in with your client about their chosen activity. This helps them stay accountable and committed to their self-care practice and also helps you identify other areas that your client may need to work on or resolve any obstacles that surface.

Honoring Resilience and Strengths

Often our clients are entrenched in their negative beliefs and pressure to meet unrealistic expectations. They tend to ignore their existing strengths and overlook their capabilities. However, when your client can reflect on past situations where they were resilient, whether big or small, they will be able to recall these times as evidence to drown out negative beliefs instead of allowing them to take hold. This increases their dissonance with their negative self-view and supports their confidence, allowing a change towards self-acceptance.

Therefore, it is important to help your client remember how resourceful they were during difficult times. When your client acknowledges their positive patterns, they will be able to use these in conjunction with their self-care activity.

CLIENT WORKSHEET: ACKNOWLEDGING POSITIVE PATTERNS

We have all faced difficult times. Can you recall a time when you were resourceful and, even though the situation was challenging, overcame it? What did you do? What did you learn? Reminders of our strengths during past stressful events can help us better manage future ones.

Objective: Identify positive patterns that support a positive self-view.
Directions: Complete the questions below to help you uncover your positive patterns. Remember not to judge any of your responses, and to complete all exercises with open curiosity.

Part 1: Resilience Recall Exercise

1. Identify specific situations that were difficult for you but you were able to overcome?

2. What specifically did you do to get through (overcome) it?

3. What are some positive traits or characteristics that you used to get through it?

4. What does this say about you from a positive perspective?

Part 2: Reflection Questions

1. What thoughts and feelings are you noticing as you're completing this worksheet?

2. How can you use your responses to questions 2, 3, and 4 in Part 1 of the worksheet to support a positive view of yourself?

3. From each situation, identify positive thoughts about yourself that you resonate with. (State in the form of I am...)

4. What happens when you repeat the positive thoughts out loud? What do you notice in your thoughts, feelings and body? How does it feel for you?

*Repeat positive thoughts while practicing daily self-care activities.

Developing self-compassion takes time and practice. Using various exercises, techniques, and tools will help your client find the ones most effective for them (Duarte et al. 2019). The next exercise is a self-compassion tool that can help your client practice being gentler towards themselves when they are self-critical. Our clients are usually empathetic, sensitive, and naturally show compassion for the people they care about. This tool can create awareness about the tone and words they use with their loved ones as opposed to the way they treat themselves. Eventually self-compassion will be part of their nature too.

RACHEL'S WORKSHEET: SELF-COMPASSION OVER CRITICISM

Identify your most common negative thoughts about yourself.

Bad things happen to me because of who I am.
It's my fault. I could've done more. I didn't do enough.
I can't help to believe that I'm not as lovable because others think that I'm fat. My stomach is fat compared to most.

What would you say to an important significant other who had this thought?
(What tone would you use?)

Loving tone: that's not true. Bad things happen all the time, not because of who you are.
Caring tone: You did what you could. It's not your fault.
Caring tone: You are lovable just the way you are.

What would you say to a child you have a strong relationship with who had this thought? (What tone would you use?)

Loving and caring soft tone: You're the best kid in the world. Bad things happen and we can learn to cope through it.
Loving caring tone. It's never a child's fault and it's not your fault.
Caring tone and loving, I know you might feel that way, but people love you no matter what.

What would you say to the child in the photo who has this thought? (What tone would you use?)

Loving and caring soft voice. I'm sorry you feel that way. You must be hurting to think that. Well, it's not true. You deserve good things.
Loving and caring tone with soft voice. It's never your fault. Your parents needed to take care of you. I'm sorry they didn't.
Caring and loving tone, I'm sorry you feel that way. I know the people who matter most love you just the way you are.

Rachel's response to Reflection Questions:

1. What feelings, thoughts and behaviors did you notice when completing this exercise?

   I noticed irritation and didn't know what I would say. But when I really imagined the people I love, it came pretty easily for me. I had thoughts that "I'm still fat and others are loveable but I'm not."

2. How can you use this tool to practice self-compassion?

   I can use it as a reminder. If I'm having a hard time with beating myself up, maybe I can write it out, and see if it works.

3. How can you use this tool to practice self-compassion?

   I can use it as a reminder. If I'm having a hard time with beating myself up, maybe I can write it out, and see if it works.

CLIENT WORKSHEET: SELF-COMPASSION OVER CRITICISM

We all have critical thoughts. But just because the eating disorder voice says them doesn't mean they're true! Turning off the eating disorder voice can feel impossible. In fact, you have probably noticed that when you try to do so, it gets louder. Although it may seem counterintuitive, one of the best ways to challenge the eating disorder voice is to be kind to yourself. Let's try it now.

Objective: Practice showing yourself self-compassion when critical thoughts pop into your head.

What you will need: A photo of yourself as a child (preferably under the age of nine)

Directions: Complete the prompts below. Remember not to judge any of your responses, and to write with open curiosity.

Part 1

Identify a self-critical thought.

What would you say to an important significant other who had this thought about themself? (What tone would you use?)

What would you say to a child you have a strong relationship with who had this thought about themself? (What tone would you use?)

What would you say to the child in the photo who has this thought about themself? (What tone would you use?)

Part 2 Reflection Questions

1. What feelings, thoughts and behaviors did you notice when completing this exercise?

2. How can you use this strategy to practice self-compassion?

3. What are some challenges you are noticing when practicing self-compassion?

Rachel's responses from the last exercise shows some progression in cultivating self-acceptance, however, body image disturbances remain problematic. Complete recovery will be difficult unless judgments about body disturbance and dissatisfaction are addressed. While Rachel understands that her negative perception is rooted from experiences in her past, her negative self-view is also fueled by her negative perception of her body. Her body dissatisfaction becomes proof of her unworthiness, fanning the flames for self-hatred.

The next chapter, foundational skill #5 *Exploring Body Neutrality and Acceptance* targets this, helping individuals explore, learn, and understand the complicated multidimensional body image disturbances tied to disordered eating.

Bibliography

Ansari, S., Asgari, P., Makvandi, B., Heidari, A., & Seraj Khorrami, N. (2020). Effectiveness of Schema Therapy in Psychological Distress, Body Image, and Eating Disorder Beliefs in Patients with Anorexia Nervosa. *Avicenna Journal of Neuro Psycho Physiology*, 7(3), 184–189 http://ajnpp.umsha.ac.ir/article-1-246-en.html.

Basile, B., Tenore, K., & Mancini, F. (2019). Early maladaptive schemas in overweight and obesity: A schema mode model. *Heliyon*, 5(9), e02361. https://doi.org/10.1016/j.heliyon.2019.e02361.

Braun, T. D., Park, C. L., & Gorin, A. (2016). Self-compassion, body image, and disordered eating: A review of the literature. *Body Image*, 17, 117–131. DOI: 10.1016/j.bodyim.2016.03.003.

Dias, B., Ferreira, C., & Trindade, I. (2020). Influence of fears of compassion on body image shame and disordered eating. Eating and Weight Disorders – Studies on Anorexia. Bulimia and Obesity, 25. 10.1007/s40519-018-0523-0.

Duarte, J., Mendes, A., Marta-Simões, J., & Ferreira, C. (2020). Striving as a paradoxical strategy to deal with fears of compassion: impact on disordered eating. *Eating and Weight Disorders – Studies on Anorexia, Bulimia and Obesity*, 25. 10.1007/s40519-019-00715-7.

Ferreira, C., Matos, M., Duarte, C., & Pinto-Gouveia, J. (2014). Shame memories and eating psychopathology: the buffering effect of self-compassion. *European Eating Disorders Review: The Journal of the Eating Disorders Association*, 22(6), 487–494. https://doi.org/10.1002/erv.2322.

Fresnics, A. A., Wang, S. B., & Borders, A. (2019). The unique associations between self-compassion and eating disorder psychopathology and the mediating role of rumination. *Psychiatry Research*, 274, 91–97. https://doi.org/10.1016/j.psychres.2019.02.019.

Geller, J. et al. (2022). Self-compassion and its barriers: predicting outcomes from inpatient and residential eating disorders treatment. *Journal of Eating Disorders*, 10(1): 114. DOI: 10.1186/s40337-022-00640-8.

Gerges, S., Hallit, S., Malaeb, D., & Obeid, S. (2022). Maladaptive Cognitive Schemas as Predictors of Disordered Eating: Examining the Indirect Pathway through Emotion Regulation Difficulties. *International Journal of Environmental Research and Public Health*, 19(18), 11620.

Joshua, P. et al. (2023). Is schema therapy effective for adults with eating disorders? A systematic review into the evidence. *Cognitive Behaviour Therapy*, 52, 1–19.

Kalika, E., Egan, H., & Mantzios, M. (2022). Exploring the role of mindful eating and self-compassion on eating behaviours and orthorexia in people following a vegan diet. *Eating and Weight Disorders: EWD*, 27(7), 2641–2651. https://doi.org/10.1007/s40519-022-01407-5.

Kelly, A. C., Carter, J. C., Zuroff, D. C., & Borairi, S. (2013). Self-compassion and fear of self-compassion interact to predict response to eating disorders treatment: A preliminary investigation. *Psychotherapy Research*, 23(3), 252–264. DOI: 10.1080/10503307.2012.717310.

Kelly, A. C., Carter, J. C., & Borairi, S. (2014). Are improvements in shame and self-compassion early in eating disorders treatment associated with better patient outcomes? *International Journal of Eating Disorders*, 47(1), 54–64. DOI: 10.1002/eat.22196.

Kelly, A. C., & Tasca, G. A. (2016). Within-persons predictors of change during eating disorders treatment: An examination of self-compassion, self-criticism, shame, and eating disorder symptoms. *International Journal of Eating Disorders*, 49(7), 716–722. DOI: 10.1002/eat.22527.

Legenbauer, T., Radix, A. K., Augustat, N., & Schütt-Strömel, S. (2018). Power of Cognition: How Dysfunctional Cognitions and Schemas Influence Eating Behavior in Daily Life Among Individuals With Eating Disorders. *Frontiers in Psychology*, 9, 2138. DOI: 10.3389/fpsyg.2018.02138.

Meneguzzo, P. et al. (2021). Associations Between Trauma, Early Maladaptive Schemas, Personality Traits, and Clinical Severity in Eating Disorder Patients: A Clinical Presentation and Mediation Analysis. *Frontiers in Psychology*, 12, 661924. DOI: 10.3389/fpsyg.2021.661924.

Neff, K. D. (2023). Self-Compassion: Theory, Method, Research, and Intervention. *Annual review of psychology*, 74, 193–218. https://doi.org/10.1146/annurev-psych-032420-031047.

Spirou, D. et al. (2022). Childhood trauma, posttraumatic stress disorder symptoms, early maladaptive schemas, and schema modes: a comparison of individuals with obesity and normal weight controls. *BMC Psychiatry*, 22, 517. https://doi.org/10.1186/s12888-022-04169-7.

Williams, B. M., & Levinson, C. A. (2020). Negative beliefs about the self prospectively predict eating disorder severity among undergraduate women. *Eating Behavior*, 37, 101384. DOI: 10.1016/j.eatbeh.2020.101384.

Yakın, D., Gençöz, T., Steenbergen, L., & Arntz, A. (2019). An integrative perspective on the interplay between early maladaptive schemas and mental health: The role of self-compassion and emotion regulation. *Journal of Clinical Psychology*, 75(6), 1098–1113. https://doi.org/10.1002/jclp.22755.

Chapter 7

Foundational Skill #5
Exploring Body Neutrality and Acceptance

Negative body image disturbance is a hallmark feature in eating disorders (Williams & Levinson 2020). It is widely known that this is an obstacle interfering with recovery and a primary indicator of potential relapse from eating disorder recovery (Keel et al. 2005). Therefore, addressing body image concerns and teaching body neutrality and acceptance is paramount. Without uncovering and addressing the underlying issues, individuals will continue to suffer from the effects of a negative body image. This is compounded by your clients' assumptions that their eating behaviors are about their dissatisfaction with their physical appearance which prevents them from dealing with their underlying issues or recognizing the function for their disordered eating.

Body image is a concept observed as the attitude, feelings, and perceptions of the individual's body size, body shape, and physical esthetics (Heider et al. 2018) and includes perceptual, cognitive-affective, and behavioral components (Ataria et al. 2021). The perceptual aspect involves how they estimate their size or weight. In the cognitive-affective area, cognitions, attitudes, and feelings towards the individual's body are taken into account. Finally, the behavioral aspect includes all behaviors that your client may engage in related to weight such as checking (for example, checking specific body parts and using this as a gauge to measure their self-worth), eating, restricting, use of laxatives, or self-induced vomiting (Zaitsoff et al. 2020).

It is not surprising that Rachel's attitude about herself is influenced by the negative perception of her body. Without addressing her negative body image, her self-acceptance and negative perception will continue to be challenging. While learning about the origins of defeatist inner core beliefs being helpful, Rachel's pessimistic thoughts persist because her negative body image supports her convictions. Let's take a look at an example of what this means.

> *"While I rubbed lotion on my skin, practicing self-care, it was hard for me not to judge the way I look. I usually avoid the mirror. But I wanted to challenge myself. It was bad. I saw a big nose. I have big thighs, a fat belly and jiggly arms—even though I was doing something nice, I couldn't let go of how big I feel. I feel like my body shows me that something is wrong with me and that no one would ever want to be with someone like me."*

In the example above, Rachel struggles to change her perception of herself even after learning about the origin of some of her beliefs. While Rachel understands and accepts how her early schemas influence how she feels, her body is a tangible reminder that she is unlovable. She recalls memories of negative judgments about her body from her mother (Oliveira et al. 2017). Therefore, it is crucial to mitigate your client's body image disturbance or at least help them understand how their concept of their body image perception operates and affects their life (Kadriu et al 2019.).

In this chapter, we explore body image dissatisfaction to help your clients understand their implicit biases about their body and how it's reinforced, address underlying issues beneath their body dissatisfaction, develop protective factors to maintain lasting eating disorder recovery, and finally enable embodiment with neutrality and acceptance. This is accomplished through exercises that bolster:

- Awareness of implicit and explicit body image biases.
- Identification of vulnerabilities and risk factors.
- Nurturing protective factors that aid in preventing relapse.

DOI: 10.4324/9781032651408-11

- Feeling comfortable in one's body.
- Self-compassion and self-acceptance.
- Body neutrality.
- Physical efficacy.
- Alternative identities not focused on body image.

Becoming Aware of Implicit and Explicit Body Image Biases

Let's begin by taking a look at implicit beliefs about body image ideals.

These are unconscious biases that have been formed through experiences and are initiated from infanthood. However, most individuals are able to recall explicit memories about their bodies at or around the time of puberty. As Rachel said:

"I first noticed that I was gaining weight when my mom told me that we have to be careful of the 'Parker thighs.' I never noticed it before, but Mom said her thighs got big when she was 12 and that I needed to be careful because the 'Parker thighs' run in the family on my maternal side. Ever since then, my thighs have been noticeable, but I can't do anything about it. I'll never have a model build with thin thighs or legs."

Negative self-evaluation in regard to body image begins during late childhood and adolescence. Self-worth is bound together with beauty ideals and associated with perceptions of success, happiness, wealth, and gratifying relationships (Hicks et al. 2022). The tripartite influence model (van den Berg et al. 2002) indicates three root factors of body dissatisfaction—parents, peers, and the media (Möri et al. 2022). This framework details the socio-cultural factors that have influence and lead individuals to evaluate their bodies unfavorably.

Let's take a look at each component in the tripartite model and how it affects and reinforces your client's beliefs about their negative body perception.

Parents

Families and parents influence the development of body image directly and indirectly. Direct influences include parent's comments about their child's body shape, weight, and eating behaviors as seen in the example with Rachel's mother. Indirect influences include parent's comments about their own bodies, weight loss goals, or remarks about others' physiques. Culturally, these criticisms have been normalized and erroneously regarded as benign since most can relate to dissatisfaction about their bodies. For example, as Rachel explained:

"Around the holidays, my entire family including my aunts would talk about how they need to lose weight. They would also put money in a pot and the person that lost the most weight, got the pot of money at the end of the year. I joined the game when I was sixteen. I didn't win. But it was a thing we did. We all bonded by the hatred of our body. Everyone would chime in and talk about what part they hated the most. I never heard anyone say anything positive about their body, ever."

Peers

Friends and peers have influence on thoughts, feelings, attitudes, and behaviors. Body discrepancy, which is defined as the perception of difference in an individual's own body as compared to the body ideal, is often experienced in adolescence. When this occurs, adolescents are at a higher risk for eating disorders, low self-esteem, depression, and low self-worth. Lack of social support from family and peers increases the risk of body dissatisfaction as it affects adolescents' self-beliefs such as their self-worth (Thompson et al. 1999).

Peers' dissatisfaction with their bodies reinforces that their friends' body dissatisfaction is normal. These beliefs are reinforced through negative body talk, self-deprecation, maladaptive eating behaviors, and interaction on social media networks. For Rachel:

"I don't have one friend that believes that their body is fine just the way it is. When I tell my friends I don't feel comfortable wearing a swimsuit to a party, they all agree and we bash our bodies and pick out the parts that bother us the most, we then compare ourselves to the girls we see on social media. We know their photos are filtered and edited, but it doesn't stop us from feeling bad about ourselves".

Media

In the past, media messages of beauty were ubiquitously plastered in magazines, billboards, and on the big screen but it was passive and overt—even then, individuals were severely impacted by their harmful effects. Subsequently, social media networks provide social interaction through likes, tagging, following, adding news feeds, picture sharing, posting, and commenting. Media and social networking sites have consequential effects on people vulnerable to body image disturbance (Möri et al. 2022) which is active and affects individuals by receiving instant confirmation after posting a negative comment about themselves by others who may feel the same way. They view other users' comments and likes as corroboration that their beliefs are true. Our clients measure and compare themselves with a continual flow of edited material, highlight reels, and filtered images that depict unrealistic standard of beauty and success—and not surprisingly are left with repugnant feelings about themselves.

Individuals who internalize beauty ideals are more likely to engage in physical appearance comparisons to assess whether they meet shared cultural standards of beauty. They peruse through others' photos and posts in order to make social comparisons, to gauge their self-worth and to assess where they may fall in the beauty hierarchy. They tend to compare themselves to others they perceive as more attractive or successful such as celebrities or those judged as meeting the standards of beauty (Lovell & Banfield 2020).

A study found that it was not the frequency or quantity of social media use, but the extent to which individuals engaged in appearance-related activities such as commenting, posting, and viewing images of themselves and their peers that predicted their levels of body dissatisfaction (Jiotsa et al. 2021). These constant comparisons lead our clients to feel discontent with themselves and to react by hyper fixating on their body and physical image in an effort to change what they perceive as unacceptable. This leads to the use of maladaptive eating behaviors such as restriction, self-induced vomiting, laxatives, or compulsive exercising.

Often individuals don't realize how these implicit and explicit messages have affected them. Rachel's next worksheet is a good example of this. The exercise will help your clients examine and explore the impact of these messages. This will generate discussion and cause clients to reflect on how these negative messages are not their own and have been learned through influence.

RACHEL'S WORKSHEET: IMPLICIT AND EXPLICIT MESSAGES ABOUT BODY IMAGE

1. What messages did you receive from your family about your body?

   My body is not okay. I needed to diet and lose weight, and it's normal.

2. What messages did you receive from your mother or father about their own bodies?

   Mom hated her body and she was unlovable because of it. Dad laughed at his body and made fun of himself. He never took himself too seriously.

3. What messages did you receive from your family about other's bodies?

   We need to be like the ones that have perfect bodies, and we do not want to be the ones that had terrible bodies. Your body makes you acceptable or not.

4. What messages did you get from your peers about their bodies?

   It's normal to bash your body. If you like your body, you're full of yourself and a narcissist.

5. What messages do you receive from the media about your body?

   If I want to live my life to the fullest and have a happy life, I need to look like the models and influencers.

6. How do you feel these messages affect your own beliefs about your body?

    Truthfully, sometimes I don't believe the messages, but everyone else does so if I don't change myself, I won't be loved and will probably not get married or someday have the family I want.

7. How can you reframe these messages using a neutral tone?

    This is hard but I guess everyone is buying into messages that aren't true? But feels they have to?

CLIENT WORKSHEET: IMPLICIT AND EXPLICIT MESSAGES ABOUT BODY IMAGE

Have you ever stopped to think about the origins of your body image beliefs? In the exercise, let's take a look at how you've been influenced and identify your learned messages about body image.

Objective: Identify origins of body image beliefs.
Directions: Complete the following questions noting both implicit and explicit messages. and then discuss with your therapist.

1. What messages did you receive from your family about your body?

2. What messages did you receive from your mother or father about their own bodies?

3. What messages did you receive from your family about other's bodies?

4. What messages did you get from your peers about their bodies?

5. What messages do you receive from the media about your body?

6. How do you feel these messages affect your own beliefs about your body?

7. How could you reframe these messages using a neutral tone?

CLIENT EXERCISE: COMPARING YOURSELF TO THE BODY IDEAL

How often have you compared yourself to someone else physically? Comparing yourself to someone else often leaves you with disappointment, feelings of shame, or worse, may even activate your negative story when you feel you don't measure up. Have you felt this way? In this exercise, we'll explore how you think about others and yourself.

Objective: Gain awareness about body image ideals

Directions: Answer the questions below to learn more about the appeal of celebrities or others that have perceived body image ideals. Then complete the post-exercise reflection questions to identify issues to address in therapy.

Identify a celebrity or someone who you possess your body image ideal? What is the body image ideal?	How do you think this person feels, thinks, and acts possessing this body image ideal?	What do you like about this body ideal and what character traits does it bring about in this person?	What character traits do you feel you would possess if you had this body image ideal?	What would be different for you if you possessed this body image ideal?

Reflection Questions: Comparing Yourself to the Body Ideal

1. In reviewing your responses, what do you feel you are really needing or wanting?

2. What are alternative ways to meet those needs or wants aside from possessing your perceived body image ideal?

As shown in the previous exercise, individuals that struggle with body image disturbance often have pre-existing insecurities that they hope will disappear by changing their physical appearance. Understanding your client's vulnerabilities and risk potential can be helpful for prevention and in assessing what your clients need at the start of eating disorder recovery.

Identifying Vulnerabilities and Risk Factors

People vulnerable to body image disturbances may have underlying struggles with depression, anxiety, tendencies towards perfectionism, lower self-esteem, and self-worth (Ganesan et al. 2018). As a result, people who are dissatisfied with their bodies are more likely to ignore their physical and mental health. They are less likely to engage in proactive behaviors such as seeking regular medical screenings and have trouble meeting dietary needs, engaging in appropriate exercise, getting enough sleep, and may engage in harmful behaviors such as smoking, diet pills, and laxative use.

This increases levels of anxiety and depression and contributes to disordered eating behaviors.

Everyone occasionally has issues with their bodies. They might wish to be taller, shorter, thinner, have a flat tummy, or muscular toned legs. However, for the average person these thoughts are usually fleeting. In contrast, those that struggle with food, weight, and body image issues can easily become obsessed with these thoughts, and this fixation can hinder all parts of their lives.

Often individuals who struggle with food and body image convince others that their life would be better if they just looked a certain way. However, as therapists we know that's not the case. Whatever your client views as their ideal body image shifts once they reach that goal. For example, if your client feels they need to lose a few pounds, once they reach that goal, another area becomes the focus for their dissatisfaction.

This is because *their eating disorder is not about their body, it's about their underlying emotions*. However, people can inadvertently reinforce this belief if they are not conscious about their own implicit biases.

Your client's dissatisfaction for their body is dictated by the way they *feel*. To illustrate this, consider why is it that some days are worse for your clients than others. For example, on Monday your client may feel okay. However, by Friday, your client can feel extremely uncomfortable and dissatisfied with their body. Their bodies haven't changed, so why is this the case? This is because your client's dissatisfaction for their bodies has a deeper meaning (Jarry 1998.). It's really not about their body, but what they feel their body represents. For instance, your client may be feeling anxious about a get together with people they haven't seen in a while. They may fear judgment by others for the weight that they gained—perceived as failure. Your client's perceived unacceptable body brings up negative emotions contributing to the dissatisfaction of their body. Therefore, the problem is not really about their body as it is about what their body represents for them.

In our next exercise, let's take a look at what lies beneath Rachel's—and your client's—dissatisfaction about their body.

RACHEL'S WORKSHEET: WHAT DOES MY BODY REPRESENT?

1. Describe your body feature(s) that you feel dissatisfied with?

   My fat belly, my big nose, my jiggly arms.

2. What about that body feature(s) bothers you the most? What feeling goes with it?

   It's round and jiggly and I feel ashamed.

3. What does this say about you (negative thought)? Complete the statement (using a negative thought) I am…

   I am an embarrassment and a failure. No one wants to love someone who is an embarrassment.

4. What is the negative statement from question 3? What would happen if this negative statement were true?

   I am an embarrassment and a failure. No one would want to be with someone like me.

5. What is currently happening in your life that is related to this negative statement?

   My boyfriend broke up with me. Why would he want to be with someone like me?

6. What do you think this body part or feature represents in relation to what is happening in your life?

   It represents my flaws and the possibility of rejection.

CLIENT WORKSHEET: WHAT DOES MY BODY REPRESENT?

In this exercise, let's take a look at what your dissatisfaction represents. Often our body represents other dissatisfactions in our life. For example, if you are feeling uncomfortable in your body because you don't like the way you look, you can ask yourself, "What else is going on today that makes me feel uncomfortable?" Or perhaps ask, "What will I be doing today that brings up feelings uneasiness for me?"

Objective: Decoding the meaning behind body dissatisfaction.
Directions: Choose a body part (feature) and then complete the following questions to decode the meaning behind your body dissatisfaction. This exercise can be completed anytime you feel dissatisfied with your body to uncover what you are feeling dissatisfied with in your current situation.

1. Describe a body feature(s) that you feel dissatisfied with?

2. What about the body feature bothers you the most?

3. What does it say about you (negative thought) that you possess the body feature? Complete the statement I am…

4. What is the negative statement from question 3? What would happen if this negative statement were true?

5. What is currently happening in your life that is related to this negative statement?

6. What do you think this body part or feature represents in relation to what is happening in your life?

In Rachel's completed worksheet, she learned that her dissatisfaction with her body represent her fear rejection. This is exacerbated for Rachel because she has recently experienced rejection—the breakup with her boyfriend. Therefore, her fear around her shortcomings leading to rejection have been confirmed. The breakup is evidence that her perceived defects need to be corrected.

Individuals project their dreams, fantasies, hopes, goals, and insecurities on their perception of the ideal body image. In the next exercise, individuals can increase consciousness and gain awareness about what they are looking to accomplish by revealing what they feel their ideal body image promises. When your client practices these exercises they will use these strategies to understand their body dissatisfaction and work on addressing what they feel they are lacking.

CLIENT EXERCISE: THE IDEAL BODY PROMISE

What do you feel will happen once you obtain the body of your dreams? In this exercise, let's find out what your ideal body image promises.

Objective: Identify your desires for your life.
Directions: Complete the following worksheet and discuss your responses with your therapist.

Identify a body feature or part that you would like to change or feel dissatisfied about.	What is your body ideal for this feature? Why is this body ideal important?	Imagine possessing the body ideal for this feature, what does this body ideal promise you?	How could you obtain this promise in another way other than through your body image?

Nurturing the Protective Factors that Aid in Preventing Relapse

We've looked at how body image perceptions are developed and the deeper representations of body dissatisfaction. Individuals can build resilience and cultivate protective factors (Tylka & Wood-Barcalow 2015) against negative messages about their body by developing the following.

- Positive body embodiment.
- Self-compassion and self-acceptance.
- Positive body and body neutrality.
- Physical efficacy.
- Other identities.

Feeling at Home in One's Body

A positive body image is a "homey" comfortable feeling in your client's bodies. They experience a feeling of purpose, a sense of autonomy, and agency in their bodies and honor their bodily needs. This motivates them to practice self-care, and have the awareness to anticipate their needs. They will ultimately be able to experience the world from the first-person viewpoint, rather than from the third-person (Burychka et al. 2021). Self-objectification involves the perception of oneself in the third person. In the previous example, Rachel perceives herself as an object that she evaluates based on physical appearance rather than from a place of embodiment— considering her body's functionality and psychological attributes. See foundational skill #1 *Connecting Mind and Body* in Chapter 3 for more exercises in developing a positive body image.

CLIENT MEDITATION: EMBODIMENT OF THE BODY

Practice the following exercise to nurture mind and body integration.

Objective: To cultivate mind and body integration.
Directions:

1. Identify a safe space to practice this exercise. This could be in your bedroom, or out in nature.
2. Scan your environment and notice how you feel in your body. Use the SUDs scale from Chapter 3 to gauge levels in your body. When you feel calm in your mind and body, close your eyes.
3. Take a breath. Notice your breath and your heartbeat. Place your hand on your chest and notice the beats. Take another breath, and scan your body from head to toe, wiggling each part of your body and noticing the movement and sensations.
4. Take another breath and focus on the air moving into your lungs and out through your mouth. Continue this breathing for ten breaths.
5. Breathe in and out with eyes closed, just observing your chest rise, and taking in air through your nose and breathing out gently through your mouth.
6. Check your SUDs level. If your SUDs level increased, continue to practice the exercise until the SUDS level is below 5.

Self-Compassion and Self-Acceptance

Self-compassion and self-acceptance emerged as protective factors for all assessed negative body image and eating disorder outcomes (Mendes et al. 2019). Studies show that self-compassion helps reduce the body shame which is commonly experienced by individuals who have disconnected from their bodies (Dias et al. 2020). See foundational skill #4 *Practicing Self-Compassion, Self-Acceptance, and Self-Care* in Chapter 6 for more practice exercises that promote self-compassion and self-acceptance.

Before moving on to the next exercise with your client, review Rachel's completed worksheet first. It sheds light on some ways that the eating disorder manifests in a client's image of themself.

RACHEL'S WORKSHEET: COMPASSION TOWARDS BODY

Identify a part of your body that you judge negatively	What is the function of this part of your body? And how does it take care of you?	Imagine the body part speaking to you in a loving way, what would it say?
My big thighs	*It allows me to bend and be flexible and walk. My thighs take care of me by keeping me up and getting me from place to place.*	*I get sad that you don't like the way I look, but I'm here for you no matter what.*
My fat belly	*It keeps me alive by storing food and keeps me strong and able to move. It takes care of me by keeping me alive.*	*I hope one day you can appreciate me. I love you no matter what and I will do my best to be efficient. Let's work together. The better you treat me, the better I treat you.*
My jiggly arms	*I need my arms to do basically everything. I would not be able to function without my arms.*	*Please don't treat me bad. There are so many people who don't even have arms and I'm glad to be yours.*

Reflection Questions

What thoughts and feelings did you notice in completing this exercise?
I was surprised because I genuinely hope I get to the place where I can feel like this towards my body.

What do you need to improve to increase self-compassion?
Keep practicing and reminding myself that I am a good person, that no one deserves to be talked to abusively.

CLIENT WORKSHEET: COMPASSION TOWARDS BODY

It is easy to get caught up in your feelings about your physical appearance. This exercise is a reminder about the function and purpose of your body and allows you to practice self-compassion towards yourself.

Objective: Develop self-compassion and self-acceptance as a protector against negative body perception.
Directions:

1. Identify parts of your body that you judge negatively.

2. Complete the boxes below by answering each question for each part of your body.

3. Continue completing the questions that follow the questions in the box.

Identify a part of your body that you judge negatively	What is the function of this body part? And how does it take care of you?	Imagine the body part speaking to you in a loving way, what would it say?

Reflection Questions

What thoughts and feelings did you notice in completing this exercise?

What do you need to improve to increase self-compassion?

Body Neutrality

Positive body image and body appreciation includes love and respect for the body. It permits appreciation of individual's uniqueness and purpose of their body. Clients that accept their bodies can embrace or at least view their bodies as neutral when there are perceived body imperfections, or variations from social and cultural standards of ideals. Your clients can connect to their mind and body and can detect their bodies' needs while rejecting unrealistic beauty ideals promoted by the media.

Positive body image does not mean that your clients are entirely content with their physical appearance. Nor does it mean that your clients are completely engrossed in body acceptance or expressed in self-absorption, or self-obsession. Further, it doesn't mean that your clients who have a positive body image are flawless at handling the bombardment of media's unrealistic standards, or relentless body shaming or body-related comments hurled their way. It just means that your client can remain neutral and possess a protective element that helps them filter out harmful messages and recognize impossible standards of beauty (Tort-Nasarre et al. 2023). They are then able to identify other unique aspects about themselves as valuable, not just their physical appearance or perceived attractiveness.

CLIENT EXERCISE: CULTIVATING A POSITIVE BODY IMAGE

It is important to recognize the uniqueness of your body. No other body is exactly the same as yours. If you close your eyes and imagine the various types of trees you have encountered in your life, you probably have noticed that each tree has its distinctive qualities that make it special. Trees are not usually judged as better or worse compared to another tree, they are just observed for their uniqueness and appreciated for what they are. This exercise allows you to recognize and appreciate your individuality.

Objective: Appreciating your uniqueness and cultivating a positive body image
Directions: Complete the questions below and discuss your responses with your therapist.

1. Describe positive aspects about your body that makes it unique or different from others.

2. Describe three life-sustaining functions that your body performs.

3. Describe three areas of your body that you appreciate that deviate from idealized messages you get from the media.

4. Describe what makes you feel beautiful, comfortable, confident, and happy.

5. What negative words did you notice as you were completing this exercise? Reframe any negative words that surfaced and replace with words that support a positive perception of your body.

One study found that older women have a higher body appreciation than younger women, and high body appreciation was found to be a protective factor for women against the negative effects of media exposure to thin models (Ferreira et al. 2017). Let's continue with body appreciation by helping our clients develop empathy for their bodies through the next exercise. See Rachel's completed exercise as an example for your clients.

RACHEL'S WORKSHEET: GRATITUDE LETTER TO BODY.

What are negative statements that you have said about your body? (Give specific examples)
You're gross! You're disgusting. No one wants to be with you. Why are you so fat and disgusting!

How have you treated your body negatively? (Give specific examples)
I've said mean things to my body. I always ignore it and say it's not deserving of food. I made my body do things it didn't want to like sleep with strange men without protection. I'm embarrassed to say more.

How have you ignored/neglected your body's needs? (Give specific examples)
The question really is, "when haven't I neglected or ignored my body's needs?" I feel too guilty to eat so I don't eat when I'm hungry. I eat too much when I'm full. I stay up to do things when I'm tired. I push myself when I'm sick.

Taking your body into consideration (separately from your mind) what feelings, and thoughts might your body be experiencing from how you've been treating your body in questions 1–3?

My body is probably feeling like it can never do anything right. It gets blamed for everything, and I've been so abusive towards my body.

Write a gratitude letter to your body incorporating your responses from questions 1–4.

Dear Body,

I never really thought about the way I treat you. I always looked at it like you're doing me wrong. I never really thought about it in the way that I've been blaming you and treating you in an extremely abusive way. I realize that I need to listen to what you need more, and I'm grateful for you being healthy even though I haven't been the best. Thank you for keeping me alive and getting me to the places I need to be. You never gave up on me even when I didn't give you the basic things you need.

With gratitude,
Rachel Parker

CLIENT EXERCISE: GRATITUDE LETTER TO BODY.

What if your body had a voice? What would your body say to you? What if your body had feelings, and thoughts? How would your body react to how you have been speaking to and treating your body? People who struggle with food, weight, and body image commonly have ignored their bodies. In this exercise, you will practice empathy towards your body to explore and understand how your body has been affected through these challenges.

Objective: Develop compassion, self-acceptance, and body appreciation.
Directions: Complete the questions then write a gratitude letter to your body incorporating the responses from the questions.

What are negative statements that you have said about your body? (Give specific examples)

How have you treated your body negatively? (Give specific examples

How have you ignored/neglected your body's needs? (Give specific examples)

Taking your body into consideration (separating from your mind) what feelings, and thoughts might your body be experiencing from how you've been treating your body in questions 1–3?

Write a gratitude letter to your body incorporating your responses from questions 1–4.

Dear Body,

With gratitude,

Physical Efficacy

Some individuals neglect physical activity due to discomfort and dissatisfaction with their bodies. For some, body image disturbance and harsh negative judgments about themselves are reasons they tend to avoid exercise in any form but lack of movement increases discontent in their bodies, making it more difficult for body acceptance. It is known that physical activity increases endorphins and dopamine levels, and promotes a sense of wellbeing. Physical efficacy is a protective factor in guarding against a negative body image and promotes eating disorder recovery.

Research indicates that it is not the type of activity makes a difference, but how individuals feel about themselves when they are participating in the activity that matters most (Marschin & Herbert 2021). When individuals engage in activities of interest, they feel more confident, effective, and stronger. This helps them feel better in their body, and they are likely to continue the past time, reinforcing positive thoughts about their body. Often clients have been critical towards themselves and have not taken the time to explore physical activities that bring them joy. (This does not pertain to individuals who struggle with compulsive exercise or use exercise as a way to compensate for eating behaviors or weight. Compulsive exercise and associated behaviors are addressed in Chapter 10, foundational skill *#7 Coping with Emotional Triggers and Building Resilience.*)

Let's explore your client's experiences with physical movement in the next exercise.

CLIENT EXERCISE: JOYFUL MOVEMENT

Everyone has their own reasons for not wanting to engage in physical activity. However, the many benefits of exercise alone are a motivation to create a routine and to help increase the positive feelings for your body. Let's explore ways to get more physical activity in your life.

Objective: To create awareness about your feelings about physical activity and to identify movement that helps you to feel positive in your body.

Directions: Complete the worksheet by answering the questions below.

---

1. What physical activity did you enjoy growing up? What made this activity enjoyable?

2. What physical activity do you currently engage in? What makes this activity enjoyable?

3. What physical activities help you to feel confident, joyous, and calm in your mind and body?

4. What part of your body keeps you from engaging in physical activity? What do you experience from this part of your body?

5. How can you incorporate daily physical activity that helps you to feel balanced and grounded in your routine?

Alternative Identities

When individuals primarily identify themselves by their physical attractiveness or appearance, it is not surprising that they struggle with issues around negative body image perception. More time will be focused on their outward appearance, and as expected they are more sensitive to others' judgments. It is imperative that individuals can identify with other qualities that make them uniquely themselves. The ability to identify with other characteristics, traits, roles, abilities, hobbies, and culture, prevents individuals from feeling constricted and trapped in their appearance as their only identity. Thus having other identities is a protective factor against body image disturbance and promotes eating disorder recovery (Vankerckhoven et al. 2023). (Identity is discussed in depth in Chapter 11, foundational skill *#9 Changing My Story*.)

In our next exercise, we explore identity and how it is connected to body image. In Rachel's earlier comments she verbalized her mother's negative judgments about their family's legs known as "Parker's thighs." Rachel's mother passed on her disapproval for this body part to Rachel. In this exercise, let's take a closer look at familial identity and body image.

This exercise creates awareness and allows your client to look at the disturbances with consciousness, developing understanding about what it means, and ultimately transforming disapproval into appreciation.

RACHEL'S EXERCISE: FAMILY IDENTITY AND BODY IMAGE

1. Describe body features that you are satisfied with. Identify family members that also share these features. How do they feel about these body features? What is your relationship with these family members?

   I like my hair, hands, and love my eyes. My grandma has the same hair color and eye color and aunts. I love Grandma. We had a great relationship. She was like a mom to me. My aunts feel neutral.

2. Describe body features that you feel neutral about. Identify family members that also share these features. How do they feel about these body features? What is your relationship with these family members?

   My feet feel neutral. I don't know anyone who has my feet, maybe my dad? I don't know. It doesn't bother me, so I never really thought about it. My Dad is just there, he's ok. I'm fine with him. We don't have a close relationship, but it's all good.

3. Describe body features that you feel dissatisfied with. Identify family members that also share these features. How do they feel about these body features? What is your relationship with these family members?

   Let's see I hate my nose, my skin, my arms, my belly and I guess my legs. These features make me feel really ugly, unwanted and like a failure. My mom has a lot of the same features. It's a love-hate relationship with my mom. I wished she was there for me. She was always inconsistent with me. I always feel like an afterthought with her. She also hates these parts.

4. What did you notice when completing this exercise? What significance, if any did how you feel about your body also reflect the way you feel about family members that share similar body features?

   I guess I feel the same way for the people who share the same features as I do about the features. I never really thought about it. That's interesting.

5. How do your family members' feelings about their shared body features influence your feelings about your body?

    I never thought they influenced me, but I did know that my mom and I felt the same about our bodies. I guess it really influenced me and it just felt normal.

6. What do you reject about the shared features? What do you appreciate about the shared body features?

    I don't want to feel how my mom feels about herself. She has always cared about what people think about her. I hate that about her and I hate that in myself. I don't know, right now I don't feel like I appreciate anything about the shared features I have with my mom. It doesn't bother me about the shared features with everyone else. Those all feel neutral. But with my mom, ugh, it disgusts me. It's just a reminder of how no one will love me.

7. What does sharing these body features with your family members say about who you are?

    With all other family members it says, I'm just a part of the family and I don't feel anything else. Sharing it with my mom, it feels like this is the reason I'm unlovable. This is the reason I'm not okay. This is the reason, I'll be alone. This is the reason I'm a failure. It says I'll never be okay.

Client Exercise: Family Identity and Body Image

Has anyone ever made comments about your physical attributes like having your father's eyes, or your mother's dimples? It's quite natural for people to make these observations when meeting someone's child for the first time. While these remarks are usually benign and neutral, hearing these reflections over time become part of your identity. Have you ever thought about features you inherited being as part of your identity and how it might influence the way you feel about your body?

Objective: Awareness of family identity and how it influences feelings towards the body.
Directions: Complete the questions in the worksheet and discuss your responses with your therapist.

1. Describe body features that you are satisfied with. Identify family members that also share these features. How do they feel about these body features? What is your relationship with these family members?

2. Describe body features that you feel neutral about. Identify family members that also share these features. How do they feel about these body features? What is your relationship with these family members?

3. Describe body features that you feel dissatisfied with. Identify family members that also share these features. How do they feel about these body features? What is your relationship with these family members?

4. What did you notice when completing this exercise? What significance, if any did how you feel about your body also reflect the way you feel about family members that share similar body features?

5. How do your family members' feelings about their shared body features influence your feelings about your body?

6. What do you reject about the shared features? What do you appreciate about the shared body features?

7. What does sharing these body features with your family members say about who you are?

As shown in Rachel's responses, Rachel has intense feelings about the body features she shares with her mother. In previous exercises, Rachel has shared some information about her attachment patterns and relationship with her emotionally unavailable mother. It is obvious that Rachel's unresolved issues with her mother are contributing to her negative sense of self and in ineffective ways of dealing with interpersonal matters.

In Chapter 8 you will help your clients to explore their attachments and relationship dynamics, and teach them the necessary tools to understand their patterns in relating to others. Without this skill, body image disturbance and eating disorder behaviors will continue as a way of coping with difficult early attachment wounds. This is foundational skill #6 *Understanding Myself in Relations to Others*.

Bibliography

Abbate-Daga, G. et al. (2010). Attachment insecurity, personality, and body dissatisfaction in eating disorders. *The Journal of Nervous and Mental Disease, 198*(7), 520–524. https://doi.org/10.1097/NMD.0b013e3181e4c6f7.

Ataria, Y., Tanaka, S. & Gallagher, S. (eds) (2021). *Body Schema and Body Image: New Directions* (online edition, Oxford Academic). https://doi.org/10.1093/oso/9780198851721.001.0001.

Burychka, D. et al. (2021). Towards a Comprehensive Understanding of Body Image: Integrating Positive Body Image, Embodiment and Self-Compassion. *Psychologica Belgica, 61*(1), 248–261. DOI: 10.5334/pb.1057.

Dias, B. S., Ferreira, C., & Trindade, I. A. (2020). Influence of fears of compassion on body image shame and disordered eating. *Eating and weight disorders: EWD, 25*(1), 99–106. https://doi.org/10.1007/s40519-018-0523-0.

Ferreira, C., Oliveira, S., & Mendes, A. L. (2017). Kindness toward One's Self and Body: Exploring Mediational Pathways between Early Memories and Disordered Eating. *The Spanish Journal of Psychology, 20*, E47. doi:10.1017/sjp.2017.50.

Ferreira, C. & Mendes C. (2020).Insecure striving as an exacerbator of the toxic effect of shame feelings on disordered eating. *Eating and Weight Disorders: EWD, 25*(3), 659–666. DOI: 10.1007/s40519-019-00668-x. PMID: 31016609.

Ganesan, S., Ravishankar, S. L., & Ramalingam, S. (2018). Are Body Image Issues Affecting Our Adolescents? A Cross-sectional Study among College Going Adolescent Girls. *Indian Journal of Community Medicine: Official Publication of Indian Association of Preventive & Social Medicine, 43*(Suppl 1), S42–S46. https://doi.org/10.4103/ijcm.IJCM_62_18.

Heider, N., Spruyt, A., & De Houwer, J. (2018). Body Dissatisfaction Revisited: On the Importance of Implicit Beliefs about Actual and Ideal Body Image. *Psychologica Belgica, 57*(4), 158–173. https://doi.org/10.5334/pb.362.

Hicks, R. E., Kenny, B., Stevenson, S., & Vanstone, D. M. (2022). Risk factors in body image dissatisfaction: gender, maladaptive perfectionism, and psychological wellbeing. *Heliyon, 8*(6), e09745. https://doi.org/10.1016/j.heliyon.2022.e09745.

Jarry, J. L. (1998). The Meaning of Body Image for Women with Eating Disorders. *The Canadian Journal of Psychiatry, 43*(4), 367–374.

Jiotsa, B. et al. (2021). Social Media Use and Body Image Disorders: Association between Frequency of Comparing One's Own Physical Appearance to That of People Being Followed on Social Media and Body Dissatisfaction and Drive for Thinness.

International Journal of Environmental Research and Public Health, 18(6), 2880. https://doi.org/10.3390/ijerph1 8062880.

Kadriu, F. et al. (2019). Characteristics and content of intrusive images in patients with eating disorders. *European Eating Disorder Review, 27*(5), 495–506.

Keel, P. K. et al. (2005). Postremission predictors of relapse in women with eating disorders. *American Journal of Psychiatry, 162*(12), 2263–2268. DOI: 10.1176/appi.ajp.162.12.2263.

Lovell, H., & Banfield, J. (2020). Implicit influence on body image: Methodological innovation for research into embodied experience. *Qualitative Research.* https://doi.org/10.1177/1468794120974150.

Marschin, V. & Herbert, C. (2021). Yoga, Dance, Team Sports, or Individual Sports: Does the Type of Exercise Matter? An Online Study Investigating the Relationships Between Different Types of Exercise, Body Image, and Well-Being in Regular Exercise Practitioners. *Frontiers in Psychology, 12*, 621272. https://doi.org/10.3389/fpsyg.2021.621272.

Monell, E., Clinton, D., & Birgegård, A. (2022). Emotion dysregulation and eating disorder outcome: Prediction, change and contribution of self-image. *Psychology and psychotherapy, 95*(3), 639–655. https://doi.org/10.1111/papt.12391.

Möri, M., Mongillo, F., & Fahr, A. (2022). Images of bodies in mass and social media and body dissatisfaction: The role of internalization and self-discrepancy. *Frontiers in Psychology, 13*, 1009792. https://doi.org/10.3389/fpsyg.2022.1009792.

Oliveira, V. R., Ferreira, C., Mendes, A. L., & Marta-Simões, J. (2017). Shame and eating psychopathology in Portuguese women: Exploring the roles of self-judgment and fears of receiving compassion. *Appetite, 110*, 80–85. DOI: 10.1016/j.appet.2016.12.012.

Thompson, J. K., Coovert, M. D., & Stormer, S. M. (1999). Body image, social comparison, and eating disturbance: a covariance structure modeling investigation. *The International journal of eating disorders, 26*(1), 43–51. https://doi.org/10.1002/(sici)1098-108x(199907)26:1<43::aid-eat6>3.0.co;2-r.

Tort-Nasarre, G. et al. (2023). Positive body image: a qualitative study on the successful experiences of adolescents, teachers and parents. *International Journal of Qualitative Studies on Health And Well-Being, 18*(1), 2170007. https://doi.org/10.1080/17482631.2023.2170007.

Tylka, T. L., & Wood-Barcalow, N. L. (2015). What is and what is not positive body image? Conceptual foundations and construct definition. *Body Image, 14*, 118–129. https://doi.org/10.1016/j.bodyim.2015.04.001.

van den Berg, P., Thompson, J. K., Obremski-Brandon, K., & Coovert, M. (2002). The Tripartite Influence model of body image and eating disturbance: a covariance structure modeling investigation testing the mediational role of appearance comparison. *Journal of psychosomatic research, 53*(5), 1007–1020. https://doi.org/10.1016/s0022-3999(02)00499-3.

Vankerckhoven, L. et al. (2023). Identity Formation, Body Image, and Body-Related Symptoms: Developmental Trajectories and Associations Throughout Adolescence. *Journal of Youth and Adolescence, 52*(3), 651–669. https://doi.org/10.1007/s10964-022-01717-y.

Williams, B. M., & Levinson, C. A. (2020). Negative beliefs about the self prospectively predict eating disorder severity among undergraduate women. *Eating Behaviors, 37*, 101384. https://doi.org/10.1016/j.eatbeh.2020.101384.

Zaitsoff, S. L., Pullmer, R., & Coelho, J. S. (2020). A longitudinal examination of body-checking behaviors and eating disorder pathology in a community sample of adolescent males and females. *International Journal of Eating Disorders, 53*(11), 1836–1843. https://doi.org/10.1002/eat.23364.

Part IV

Teaching Intrapersonal and Interpersonal Skills for Recovery

Foundational Skill #6
Understanding Myself in Relation to Others

Rachel: "I don't trust my mother. She was never there for me as kid. I don't want to look like her. I don't want to be like her. I tell myself I don't care, but it still bothers me. I haven't ever told anyone because I just don't trust anyone."

It is known that individuals that struggle with eating issues have higher rates of insecure attachment (Kuipers et al. 2017) and research has shown that insecure attachment is a risk factor for the emergence of problematic eating, body image, and weight concerns (Keating et al. 2013).

When individuals feel insecure in their relationships, it severely affects and undermines their wellbeing in many areas. Often people are not aware that many of their challenges are part of their insecure attachment style (Cortés-García et al. 2019), including:

- **Adverse Childhood Experiences (ACES):** ACES occurs in the great majority of individuals with insecure attachment and with eating disorders (Monteleone et al. 2020). It is important to assess for childhood trauma when conducting your client's biopsychosocial assessment during the intake process. In severe cases of unresolved trauma, it is important to refer your client to a specialist that works with trauma if you are not informed in this area.
- **Interpersonal and Relational Difficulties:** Exhibiting either hyperactivating or deactivating strategies to avoid relational stress, which prevents them from acquiring the social skills necessary to thrive and receive support in their relationship.
- **Dysfunctional Emotion Regulation:** Maladaptive coping strategies include suppressing or emphasizing their responses to their emotions by binge eating, restriction of food, purging, or compulsive overexercising. In addition, they often struggle with determining what they are feeling and the origins of their emotion.
- **Body Dissatisfaction:** Prone to internalizing social standards such as the ideal body type, striving towards acceptance and approval from others. They are dissatisfied when their body goals are not obtained (Abbate-Daga et al. 2010).
- **Neuroticism:** Exhibiting neurotic personality characteristics such as negative affect, affective instability and anxiety. These traits naturally affect interpersonal relationships specifically when individuals are unaware of how this affects them.
- **Maladaptive Perfectionism:** Likely to be overly self-critical, and because they often feel unworthy, unlovable, and hopelessness, they rely on perfectionistic tendencies to strive for unrealistic achievements including with their own body.
- **Reduced Mindfulness Capacity:** Difficulty staying present and typically unable to be fully aware of their present reality. They have a tendency for anxiety and worry about future situations, such as future abandonment from others. They may also avoid the issues that are occurring in the present, such as interpersonal conflict, or paying attention to hunger and fullness cues.
- **Comparing Themselves:** Excessive comparison to others as a way to assess self-worth and value. This leads to negative self-perceptions, which leads to feelings of shame, anxiety, worthlessness, and overly critical and perfectionistic tendencies. This promotes dysfunctional eating behaviors because often the comparisons have to do with self-image.

DOI: 10.4324/9781032651408-13

- **Commitment to Therapy:** Committing to therapy is challenging. They abandon therapy more frequently and tend to change therapists more often. They are sensitive to rejection and often will avoid uncomfortable topics or fixate on the other person searching for flaws so that they can discontinue treatment. Building rapport and a therapeutic alliance are important aspects when working with this attachment type.

Self-Awareness in Relationships

With the repercussions of an insecure attachment impacting so many facets of your client's life, helping your clients understand themselves in relation to other people is crucial to their recovery, and this chapter will show you how.

Your client may have difficulty in interpersonal relationships but don't know why. Their maladaptive skills learned in their family of origin negatively affect their current relationships—and yet they may not recognize that their dysfunctional patterns exist. Without the awareness and understanding about how their family environment influences their interactions, individuals can experience intense emotional distress, activating severe hopelessness. Frequently, they do not have the coping strategies to work through these feelings, and may become flooded with discomfort and confusion and develop maladaptive techniques (Lenzo et al. 2021) (food behaviors, self-harm) to avoid the magnitude of the impact it has on them.

Because of their insecure attachment style, they view themselves and their interpersonal situations from a negative and conflicted lens (Ivanova et al. 2017). This causes challenges in their relationships. However, when individuals are aware of their ineffective tendencies—patterns in relating—they can make the necessary changes to heal old attachment wounds. They will have the opportunity to recognize ineffective patterns and emotional triggers so that they can practice relating in healthier ways. It is also important that they learn how to cope with emotional triggers. Building resilience is paramount to long lasting eating disorder recovery and is closely tied to insecure attachment. This will be addressed in depth in the next chapter.

In this chapter, your client will explore, identify and practice through exercises and worksheets:

- Attachment history: Understanding, recognizing, and giving themselves what they need.
- Attachment style: Understanding their emotional and behavioral reactions and coping tendencies.
- Interpersonal and romantic relationship patterns: Recognizing their attachment tendencies in relationships.
- Interpersonal problems and social functioning challenges.

Let's take a look at attachment.

Exploring Attachment History with Your Client

Children need to know they are safe, protected, and cared for in order to survive, thrive, and feel secure. Therefore, they are inherently motivated towards connection with primary attachment figures. In the crucial first year of life, according to Bowlby (Bosmans et al. 2022), infants develop emotional bonds with their main caregiver. "Internal working models" are representations about themselves and the social world. The availability and accessibility of caregivers (Monteleone et al. 2017) determines the extent of these mental representations and become the foundation for their attachment template.

Secure and healthy relationships provide emotional support, and comfort during stressful times, and children internalize their daily interactions and experiences with their caregivers. When significant adult figures are emotionally available, responsive, and sensitive to a child's needs they form "positive working models." Children then operate from a positive working model of the self, such as seeing themselves as "worthy of care." They feel that they matter—and perceive others as a reliable source of support (Cortés-García et al. 2019).

However, when adults are inconsistent, unreliable, and unresponsive, then negative working models are activated (Lenzo et al. 2022). Children internalize "negative working models," experiencing themselves as, "not worthy of care" and as "unacceptable" (Gagliardi 2021).

Rachel: "I don't remember my mom ever really being there for me. I just always felt like a burden to her. She always had this face where she looked irritated or angry anytime she looked at me."

In the example with Rachel, children who have a relationship with an unsympathetic attachment figure develop the belief that they are an "unworthy" and an "unlovable person", while a child with an empathetic parent, will develop beliefs about being a "lovable, worthy person."

Let's explore and learn more about your client's attachment and the important figures that influenced your clients' lives. This will help your client learn more about themselves, their relationships, and where some of their negative beliefs about themselves and other people originate. Doing so will help them understand themselves better so they can practice self-compassion. They can gain clarity about their own needs and can learn to develop healthy attachments with other people, no longer needing to rely on their eating disorder as their attachment.

We start with Rachel again, as the answers on her completed worksheets may be viewed as a typical example of an eating disorder origin story.

RACHEL'S WORKSHEET: ATTACHMENT FIGURES

1. Who were significant caregivers in your childhood? Describe the relationship.

   My father was mostly working and didn't really have much to say. He kept himself busy, so I didn't really look at him as an attachment figure. Granny was a big part of my life as a kid. She took care of me when my mom was working. She kept me safe and fed and all that, but she didn't understand me. She never asked me if I was okay. But she would always tell me not to let things bother me. I wanted my mother to be a bigger part of my life than she could be. I wanted her to come to my school events, but she never did. No one ever showed up for me. I don't know if I can say my mom was an important attachment figure in my life. I feel like she is because of the way that she, not being there still affects me.

2. Describe a time when you felt completely loved, supported, or cared for by one of these individuals.

   This is so sad but it's true. I have never felt completely loved or cared for by anyone. Not from any adult in my life, and definitely not from my attachment figures. The closest thing I've felt was some support from my granny and my dad said some nice things but never felt unconditional support or love.

3. Describe a time when you felt unloved or disrespected by one of these caregivers.

   I always feel unloved and uncared for by my mother. I feel like I am always a burden, after-thought or just an irritation to her. I can't tell you one specific time because it's all the time. One example is she constantly and consistently lies to me. She makes promises, and always breaks them and then denies she made that promise.

4. How do you feel your experiences, interactions, and relationship with these caregivers affect your beliefs about yourself? What feelings, thoughts, and beliefs do you have about yourself as result of your relationships with them?

   I don't have any good thoughts about myself. I always feel like I'm bothering someone when I'm even asking a simple question. I feel like a huge burden. I feel unworthy, unlovable, undeserving and I'm afraid. I don't trust myself. I don't trust my feelings, thoughts, and I doubt myself a lot.

CLIENT WORKSHEET: ATTACHMENT FIGURES

Who was there for you when you were a child? Which adults were responsive to your emotional needs, showed you comfort, made you feel loved and valuable? Exploring these early relationships can help you understand more about yourself, as well as the patterns in relationships you have now.

Objective: Explore important caregiver figures and how these relationships impact you today.
Directions: Complete the questions below and share with your therapist.

1. Who were significant caregivers in your childhood? Describe the relationship.

2. Describe a time when you felt completely loved, supported, or cared for by one of these individuals.

3. Describe a time when you felt unloved or disrespected by one of these caregivers.

4. How do you feel your experiences, interactions, and relationship with these caregivers affect your beliefs about yourself? What feelings, thoughts, and beliefs do you have about yourself as result of your relationships with them?

A Negative Working Model

Rachel's example shows how she felt neglected, emotionally unsupported, and deceived by her mother. Rachel recognizes how the lack of care she received from her mother impacts how she views herself which helps Rachel to understand where her negative feelings started. Without this understanding, Rachel will continue to displace her negative feelings, such as being unlovable and unworthy, on to something else, such as her physical body.

In an ideal scenario, primary caregivers would naturally provide the necessary emotional support, security, safety, and love to their children. Caregivers would have resolved most of their own childhood pain, and be available to provide the attunement and mirroring that their children need (De Groot & Rodin 1998). Unfortunately, this is rarely the case. Many parents are challenged by their own disruptive attachment patterns that have prevented them from providing love and care to their offspring.

Therefore, although Rachel would have liked for her mother to have acknowledged her absence and apologized, these corrective behaviors alone will not help Rachel heal from her internalized "negative working model." The corrective actions may help Rachel start healing her feelings towards her mother—however, it will not change the way Rachel views and feels about herself.

Rachel's child-self did not get what she emotionally needed. Her child part internalized painful, emotional, implicit, experiences of aloneness and fear. Without healing, the emotional child part does not just disappear when one becomes an adult. The implicit processes are stored and remain dormant until triggered by distressing events that activate the pain of the wounded child. When it is activated, the adult is immediately flooded and overwhelmed by emotional distress and self-defeating thoughts.

Because Rachel has been viewing herself through a negative lens, she often feels unworthy and undeserving. She emotionally neglects herself, and frequently emotionally abandons herself, re-enacting the emotional neglect and abandonment she experienced as a child. While she has a deep fear that others will treat her in this way, her propensity in behaving this way towards herself is entrenched.

Rachel: "When I'm sad and feel hurt by others I care about, I eat and try to ignore what I'm feeling. I get angry at myself and call myself really mean names. Then I just tell myself I don't deserve to be cared for."

The next exercise helps your client to identify their past unmet needs. When your client has clarity about their needs, they can practice loving actions towards themselves instead of seeking out others to take on those responsibilities. People who have an insecure attachment style may have difficulty differentiating between real and unrealistic expectations in relationships (Mason et al. 2022). They need to learn to distinguish between what they internally need and recognize that while others can support them they are ultimately responsible for their own feelings, and actions.

In this case, in order for Rachel to heal and to correct old patterns she has to identify what she needed and didn't receive as a child (Monteleone et al. 2021). Next, she will need to identify how those unmet needs affect her in her current life. Lastly, she will have to practice (as the adult) giving herself the things she felt she did not receive to her child self. Rachel will need to learn to be her own mother—the mother she didn't experience growing up.

Rachel's Worksheet: Your Attachment Needs

1. Describe your relationship with an early caregiver.

    My relationship with my mom affected me a lot growing up. It's changed a lot, but only because I don't care as much anymore. When I was a kid, age 3-12. I cared a lot. She was never there and would lie a lot to me. In my teen years, we just fought a lot and I was angry at her, but she just thought I was a problem, so I gave up. Now as an adult. I know how my relationship with her has affected all my romantic relationships.

2. Describe what you feel was missing from your relationship.

    My relationship with my mom was missing everything required to have a trusting, loving caring relationship, love, trust, understanding, time, patience, everything a mother represents was missing in the relationship. It probably would have been better for me if I didn't have a mother. The worst part was having a mother that didn't care about you. That sends a big message.

3. Describe what your ideal relationship with your caregiver would have looked like.

    Honestly, I don't think I wanted that much. I didn't have an unrealistic version of a great mom. My ideal mom would've just been for a mom that cared, loves me, is attentive, gave me time, was consistent, let me know I matter and the needs I had mattered. When I would cry and let her know I was sad and needed her, that it didn't just fall to deaf ears.

4. What are some feelings, thoughts or behaviors you wish your caregiver would have considered in your relationship?

    I wish she would have considered her decision to have a child. She wasn't ready for a child, then she should have never had one. I wish she would have just considered her children and how her behaviors and selfishness affected everyone.

5. On the chart, make a list of needs that you wish your caregiver would have met for you. Then, list the actions they could have taken to satisfy your need. In the third column, indicate what you could do for yourself to meet your need. Finally, in the last column, indicate specific behaviors you can practice so that you can be there for yourself.

What did you need?	List the actions your caregiver could have taken to meet your needs.	How can you meet this need for yourself today?	What specific behaviors can you practice when you are needing what you listed in the first column?
To know that I matter.	*Make time for me, tell me I mattered, show me I mattered by doing things I care about. Show up for me.*	*I know I have to tell myself I matter and show up for myself. I need to care about what happens to me.*	*Acknowledge my feelings when I feel sad. Give myself time, such as take a break or ask myself what I need, like a walk, or a massage.*
To know that she would always be there.	*I wish that mom would've followed through on her promises. I wish she was on time and to pick me up. I wish she was always dependable and reliable.*	*I have to keep my word to myself. I have to always be dependable and reliable for myself when I'm in need.*	*When I feel down. I need to be consistent and reliable. I cannot just check out and ignore my feelings. I need to reach out to others or do things that help me feel better.*
To have a relationship with my mother.	*I wish my mom would've treated me like her daughter. Do special mother daughter things together like everyone else.*	*I guess I have to treat myself like I wanted my mom to have treated me. I guess my relationship with myself needs to be treating myself in special ways.*	*I definitely need to talk to myself in a much kinder way. I can talk to myself the way I wanted my mom to talk to me. It's like have compassion. I've been practicing it, so it is getting easier.*

CLIENT WORKSHEET: YOUR ATTACHMENT NEEDS

When you were an infant, you trusted your caregiver to provide what you needed, even when you didn't know exactly what you did need. This trust continued as you became a child. However, if a caregiver didn't give you what you need, you may have lost trust in your caregivers. Now, the gift of being older is learning to recognize those unmet needs, and how those unmet needs are impacting you today. This insight can then empower you to meet your own needs—because ultimately, we are the only ones that know exactly what we need, and how it needs to be given to us.

Objective: Gain an understanding of your core needs and identify how unmet needs impact you today. Practice giving those needs to yourself.

Directions:

Think about your childhood. Think about the adults that you would seek comfort from.
    How would these adults respond to your needs?

1. Choose a caregiver that you feel had significantly impacted you.
2. With the caregiver in mind, answer the questions below.

---

1. Describe your relationship with an early caregiver.

2. Describe what you feel was missing from your relationship.

3. Describe what your ideal relationship with your caregiver would have looked like.

4. What are some feelings, thoughts or behaviors you wish your caregiver would have considered in your relationship?

5. On the chart, make a list of needs that you wish your caregiver would have met for you. Then, list the actions they could have taken to satisfy your need. In the third column, indicate what you could do for yourself to meet your need. Finally, in the last column, indicate specific behaviors you can practice so that you can be there for yourself.

What did you need?	List the actions your caregiver could have taken to meet your needs.	How can you meet this need for yourself today?	What specific behaviors can you practice when you are needing what you listed in the first column?

Unblending from the Child Self

Often clients are resistant to and challenged by the thought of having to be responsible for their own emotional needs because they didn't receive what they should have in childhood. It is developmentally appropriate for young children to be egocentric. Young children need to feel loved, cared for, and know that they matter. Therefore, for adults that haven't worked through their attachment challenges, being unable to provide for their own needs is considered evidence that they are not important or lovable.

Rachel: "That worksheet and exercise was hard. Honestly, I know I've come a long way but as I was completing the worksheet, I was thinking, 'Why the heck do I have to do all the work, why can't someone else just come and do this for me?' It just feels so hard. And sometimes, the negative voice kicks in and says, 'Because you don't deserve for others to do this for you. But I completed the worksheet anyway, so I know it's getting a little better.'"

Therefore, it is important for your client to practice accessing and connecting to parts other than the child self. When individuals have issues with unresolved attachment, their child self tends to take charge. This child part engages in a reactive way and often gets overwhelmed by intense emotions and can be resistant to taking on responsibility for themselves. For example, we would not expect any five-year-old to know how to give themselves emotionally what they need—nor do we expect them take on the responsibilities of an adult.

Although your client is an adult, when their child part has been activated they are emotionally operating at a younger age and can feel stuck and have trouble giving themselves what they need. They can emotionally feel like a five-year-old.

This next exercise will help your client connect to parts of themselves that they may not normally think about or know exist. This powerful visualization helps your client access and connect to their nurturing adult part.

Clinician note: People struggling with issues with attachment naturally have the urge to nurture or take care of things that are important to them—such as their loved ones, their personal possessions, animals, or plants. However, they struggle with taking care of their emotional selves.

Client Exercise: Connecting to Your Inner Nurturer

Have you ever thought of yourself as being made up of different parts? Like maybe you have an inner athlete who loves being sporty, or an inner nerd who likes nothing better than to curl up with a book? In this exercise, you will explore your *inner nurturer,* which you can think of as a mother or father or another caregiver figure, and your *inner child,* which represents you when you were little.

Objective: Learn to access and connect to parts of the self (in this case the inner nurturer) in order to take care of unmet emotional needs.

What you will need:

- Quiet room.
- Drawing paper.
- Pens.
- A Photo of yourself (age range infant to nine years).
- At least 30 minutes of quiet time.

Directions:

1. Practice before bed particularly if you have had a challenging day.

2. Close your eyes and visualize your inner nurturer.

3. What does she physically look like? (It can take any form. This figure could be a person, a feeling, an impression, abstract colors or shapes.)

4. Once you have clarity about what your inner nurturer feels and looks like, imagine your inner nurturer meeting your inner child. Use the photo of your young self to help you visualize.

5. If you are experiencing difficulty with connecting to your inner child part, reflect on what your inner child may have been feeling, thinking, or needing when the photo was taken.

6. Imagine your inner nurturer asking your inner child what it needs. Refer back to the exercise "Attachment Needs" and practice addressing the needs from the nurturer to your child self.

7. Complete the questions below and share with your therapist.

8. Practice this exercise nightly for 30 days.

---

1. What does your inner nurturer look, feel, and sound like?

2. Draw an image of your inner nurturer.

3. What do you most connect with about your inner nurturer?

4. What is the child in the photo feeling, thinking, needing, or wanting?

5. Review the list of specific wants and needs (from "Attachment needs" worksheet # 5).

6. What was the visualization process like for you? What did you notice? What were challenges? What was unexpected?

7. What can you work on in your next visualization?

Understanding Your Client's Attachment Style

Attachment styles encompass your client's cognitive and emotional perceptions of themselves and impact their feelings, thoughts, behaviors, attitudes, and decisions when in a relationship with others. These styles were shaped by repeated interactions with important caregivers, forming their sense of security, their strategies for coping, and the structures in place for affect regulation and their ability to recognize attachment needs. Helping your client identify their attachment style helps them to understand themselves better. In turn, they can better understand their tendencies when interacting with others.

Both anxious and avoidant styles are considered insecure attachments: securely attached individuals exhibit low levels of anxiety and avoidance. Attachment styles reflect their beliefs, trustworthiness, and supportiveness with patterns of interpersonal perceptions, behaviors, and strategies for affect regulation.

Secure

People with a secure attachment style have received responsive and available support from primary caregivers. They have a positive view about themselves, and believe that others are available, and show adaptive emotion regulation (Kaurin et al. 2022).

In relationships they are comfortable with depending on and seeking intimacy in their partner. They are able to feel emotionally connected with their partner even when their partner isn't present. In stressful situations, they seek interpersonal comfort and feel emotionally connected to their support system. They are trusting, have an internalized secure base, a coherent sense of self, the ability to forgive and give others the benefit of the doubt, and can recognize the value of relationships in their own growth and development.

Anxious

These are individuals who received inconsistent or unpredictable care, resulting in high attachment anxiety. They developed negative working models that lead them to believe they are unworthy and unlovable and therefore have an overall negative self-view. However, they developed a conflicting working model with others, in that they are hopeful that their significant other can provide care and security, but they are not confident. These individuals are hypervigilant and suspicious of others' intentions because of their rejection sensitivity. They are constantly needing reassurance and evidence that they are loved by their partners (Kaurin et al. 2022).

They tend to utilize hyperactivating strategies (such as clingy, controlling, or coercive behaviors) and hypervigilance when threatened in stressful interpersonal situations. They experience attachment anxiety worrying about being abandoned and underappreciated by their partners. Research shows that attachment anxiety is positively associated with eating disorders and regulation of anxious attachment is associated with body image concerns (Lev Arey et al. 2023). This attachment style tends to use food as a way to cope with anxiety so they tend to struggle with emotional or binge eating.

Avoidant

These individuals had caregivers that may have been cold or rejecting. Therefore, they have difficulty trusting others in an intimate relationship and expect their partners to be unavailable and undependable when they may need emotional support. They typically avoid intimacy and seek out independence and self-reliance (Girme et al. 2018). Therefore, most individuals who tend to be restrictive towards food have an avoidant attachment style. They not only avoid food—they also tend to avoid relationships.

Avoidant attachment types utilize deactivating strategies such as denying their attachment needs, being compulsively self-reliant, and other behaviors that keep others at a distance. They have negative working models and perceive others as emotionally unavailable. They fear being vulnerable and are highly sensitive to rejection (Kaurin et al. 2022.). They strive for autonomy and to maintain control at all times when in relationships. They can have high esteem—mostly because they can be extremely self-reliant and have a tendency towards perfectionism. However, they can also be highly self-critical with a negative self-perception (Mason et al. 2017). They use coping strategies such as emotional suppression, avoidance motivation, and emotional withdrawal. People who have avoidant attachment style are more vulnerable to using excessive exercise as a coping mechanism for emotions and to manage their body image concerns (Lev Arey 2023).

Therapist Tip:

- *For this exercise, please go over attachment styles with your client before having them complete this worksheet.*

RACHEL'S WORKSHEET: WHAT'S YOUR ATTACHMENT STYLE?

---

1. What do you feel your predominant attachment style is and what have you observed in yourself to come to that conclusion?

    My attachment is definitely anxious when I was younger and when I first meet people. But then, once I get to know them better, I tend to become more avoidant. I don't want people to know I care or that I'm hurt. But I am dying inside, and I use food and other things to cope. My negative thoughts get really strong when I feel rejected and I am constantly depressed.

2. How do you feel your attachment style affects your feelings, thoughts, attitudes, decisions, and behaviors about yourself?

    It affects my mood. I'm up and down and depends on how well my relationships are doing. I am mostly negative about myself. I do have pockets where I'm okay but that's only when people are interested in me. When they are not interested, I feel horrible and worthless, unlovable. I make terrible decisions because of my attachment style. I logically know it's not the best for me, and I do it anyway. It's like a reflex.

3. How do you feel your attachment style affects your relationships with others?

    I don't trust others. I usually stay by myself and tell myself no one matters and try to stay focused on what I'm doing. I'm never the first to reach out nor do I invite people to things. I'm afraid they will say no. So I just wait for their invites. I'm hurt but don't show it when I people forget about me.

4. Describe a time when your style of attachment created conflict with family, friends, co- workers, or the community?

    It's never really created conflict because I'm usually avoidant. I only show my anxiety traits to the one significant other that is closest to me. With everyone else, I am avoidant, and they have no idea I am bothered.

5. How do you feel your attachment style affects your romantic relationships? Describe a time when your style of attachment created conflict with your partner.

    Every single time. Now I know that every single relationship ended because of my style of attachment. I either overreact or made the wrong choices in a partner. This is still because of my attachment style. One good example, in the last relationship, we got into an argument, and I felt so anxious. I was way clingy and called his phone like 100 times in a roll. He just ignored me and turned his phone off. I don't like feeling out of control like that. Every single person has broken up with me because of my behaviors.

6. How do you feel your attachment style affects your relationship with food, weight, and body image?

    When we fight, I tend to stop eating or I cannot stop eating. Also, I feel undesirable because of my body and am always on a diet so that I can find myself a relationship so I don't end up alone

Client Worksheet: What's your Attachment Style?

You probably have never thought about your particular attachment style when it comes to relationships—with others and with food. So, let's reflect for a moment on significant relationships in the past. Doing so will give you insight into your habits, their origins, and how they're playing out for you today.

Objective: Identify your attachment tendencies and how it affects you.
Directions: Complete the following questions to explore your attachment tendencies. Talk about your responses with your therapist.

1. What do you feel your predominant attachment style is and what have you observed in yourself to come to that conclusion?

2. How do you feel your attachment style affects your feelings, thoughts, attitudes, decisions, and behaviors about yourself?

3. How do you feel your attachment style affects your relationships with others?

4. Describe a time when your style of attachment created conflict with family, friends, co- workers, or the community?

5. How do you feel your attachment style affects your romantic relationships? Describe a time when your style of attachment created conflict with your partner.

6. How do you feel your attachment style affects your relationship with food, weight, and body image?

Relational Attachments to Food

Rachel: "Food is always there for me. Yes, I have a love-hate relationship with it. When I'm having a hard day at work, the first thing that usually comes to mind is I can't wait to get home and just put a movie on and just eat."

It is common for people who struggle with disordered eating to have a similar attachment style to food. For some, food may have been a stable consistent presence. It may have represented security or unconditional love. For many, dealing with the challenges of relationships, food becomes a replacement. Therefore, many who struggle with eating tend to isolate while engaging in food behaviors. To counter this behavior, since a sense of belonging is a basic human need, meaningful connection with others is an important aspect of lasting eating disorder recovery.

The caregiver's ability to respond to the attachment needs of their offspring is a direct reflection of the caregiver's sensitivity—defined as how appropriately and efficiently the parent is able to detect and assuage the child's needs. Therefore, it would be beneficial for your client to learn how their family system and structure affects and reinforces their interpersonal patterns—and how their family dynamics also can reinforce their dysfunctional eating behaviors.

Looking at Your Client's Family Systems and Structure

The family system and the way it functions plays an essential role in the maintenance of dysfunctional eating behaviors. While eating disorders can develop at any age, adolescents are the most vulnerable age group for the onset of an eating disorder. Studies have identified that those from families that have emotional disengagement, less emotional closeness, lack warmth and emotional support, have low affective expression, and excessive interpersonal dependence are more at risk in developing problems with eating (Gander et al. 2015).

Studies have shown that people diagnosed with anorexia have described their families as conflict avoidant. In contrast, individuals diagnosed with bulimia reported highly conflictual families, while people who suffer from binge eating have poor expression, ineffective communication, and poor family cohesion (Erriu et al. 2020).

It was identified that these families have unspoken agreed-upon rules. Family rules included topics such as restriction of talking about topics that bring emotional discomfort to the family, restriction to the expression of thought, and feelings or topics about members of the family that could cause any other member to feel uncomfortable. These rules increase the risk of developing pathological eating behaviors and is worsened when there are also restrictive rules regarding food.

RACHEL'S WORKSHEET: UNDERSTANDING MY FAMILY SYSTEM

The nuclear family has significant influence on how we interact with others. From our family of origin, not only did we learn how to relate with one another, we also learned how to tolerate one another. Every family has its strengths and shortcomings. How did your family system impact you?

Objective: Gain awareness about your early family system and how it influences you today when relating with others.

Directions: Take a few minutes to reflect on your nuclear family then complete the questions below.

1. How did your family members deal with conflict with one another?

   Everyone yells at each other. Then they ignore each other. Then no one ever acknowledges they were wrong or apologizes. Then when it blows over after a week or so, people slowly start talking again. The topic is never brought back up. Then it starts over if there is another conflict.

2. How did your family members show they care for one another?

   I guess on holidays they spend time together. And maybe we share food but that's pretty much it.

3. What coping methods or behaviors have you noticed that your family members use to deal with their emotions?

   No females show their emotions. If they're feeling something, they leave the house or they stay in their bedrooms. I guess they isolate. I've watched my mom clean the entire house angrily and throw away my personal items while she was at it. No one dare say anything about it. The males would break things, slam doors, and stomp around. They are aggressive.

4. What have you noticed about your family that you find unique to other families?

   I remember thinking as a kid, no one fights as much as our family. The fights were aggressive. Things were thrown, and it got physical a lot of times too. Not with me, but with the other family members. I would hear it but not see it because I would be under a blanket in my bedroom, too afraid to come out. Every holiday was ruined because of fighting. I learned not to get excited about happy things, because it would be ruined or cancelled. It never failed.

5. Describe what safety would feel and look like in your family.

   Consistency. People following through on what they say. People looking out for each other rather than every man for himself. And peace. If we had disagreements and it was ok to just talk about it without aggression or bullying tactics. Everyone including my parents would leave when there was conflict. I was always alone and scared.

6. What were some family rules that were known to all members (spoken and unspoken)?

    Do not have any feelings. Do not ever talk family problems with anyone. Do not ever hold anyone accountable for their poor actions. Never share your sadness and disappointments or call anyone out for lying. Lying was okay by everyone. Telling the truth brings shame. And you get punished for telling the truth. Always cover up bad actions from others even if it hurts you.

7. How do you feel your family system has impacted you in your socially and in your romantic relationships?

    I have a hard time finding healthy people. I am drawn and feel more comfortable around people who tend to take advantage of me or do not have my best interest at heart. I'm afraid to show who I really am. I always feel that people don't want to get to know me. I get bored and have no interest in people who seem stable.

Client Worksheet: Understanding My Family System

The nuclear family has a significant influence on how we interact with others. Not only do we learn how to relate with one another—we also learn to tolerate one another since we did not choose the members of our clan. Every family has its strengths and shortcomings. How did your family system impact you?

Objective: Gain awareness about your family system and how it influences you when relating with others.
Directions: Take a few minutes to reflect on your nuclear family then complete the questions below.

1. How do your family members deal with conflict with one another?

2. How do your family members show they care for one another?

3. What coping methods or behaviors have you noticed that your family members use to deal with their emotions?

4. What have you noticed about your family that you find unique to other families?

5. Describe what safety would feel and look like in your family.

6. What were some family rules that were known to all members (spoken and unspoken)?

7. How do you feel your family system has impacted you in your relationships or socially?

From Family System to Intimacy

Rachel: "I always knew my family wasn't perfect. I knew it was dysfunctional. What I didn't realize was that my family system taught me everything I know about how to be in relationships. It taught me how to love, fight, and care (or not) for each other. I guess that's why I've never had a healthy romantic relationship."

The family system and your client's attachment style influence all relationships. Even when individuals are aware of their dysfunctional tendencies and decide to make a conscious effort to change ineffective interactions learned in their family, their decision to do that is still influenced by their nuclear family.

Therefore, the family system has a significant impact on interpersonal and romantic relationships. Let's help your client explore and understand how their family system has influenced them in interpersonal and romantic relationships.

Identifying Interpersonal and Romantic Relationship Patterns

Those who have an insecure attachment style are more challenged in interpersonal and romantic relationships. For example, many studies have shown that insecure patterns of attachment are connected to a strong sense of loneliness (Troisi et al. 2005). This is believed to be the case because an individual's inner working model for attachment is biased by a filter of their own existing interpersonal beliefs and expectations. Therefore, insecure attachment can threaten quiet moments of aloneness to become an intolerable situation of loneliness.

The biased filter with which individuals with insecure attachment experience situations are a challenge for relationships.

Rachel: "My boyfriend and I fought daily. He said he couldn't be with me any more because I couldn't see things for what it is, and I only see things the way I want to see them. I don't really understand what he means because that's just the way I feel. He said I drain his energy. It just confirms that I'm not worthy. I get so confused because other days I feel like he completely understands me, and I've never felt so loved. I can feel okay."

The cumulative effects of these relationships can initiate changes in the individual's working model over time since it is considered a dynamic system. According to Bowlby (Cassidy et al. 2013), the inner working model of attachment is not determined but is pliable and can be changed, for example through new resourceful relational experiences. On days when individuals feel more accepted by their romantic partners, they reported lower levels of anxiety and avoidance. Therefore, romantic partners become primary attachment figures in adulthood and can affect an individual's mental health and welfare. When the relationship is stable and positive it may help individuals develop into a more secure style of relating (Kirby et al. 2015).

Let's explore your client's interpersonal patterns.

CLIENT WORKSHEET: EXPLORING INTERPERSONAL PATTERNS

Have you ever noticed that misunderstandings and disagreements have similar themes? We often don't realize how our patterns of relating are affecting our relationships. However, we can explore our relationships and identify the ineffective patterns that consistently show up so that we can practice new ways of relating.

Objective: Recognize ineffective relational patterns and practice new ways of relating.
Directions: Complete the following questions and share with your therapist.

1. Describe your relationship with your closest friend.

2. Describe a significant relationship with a romantic partner.

3. Describe your worst fear in your relationships. How do you go about preventing this from happening?

4. Describe any interpersonal patterns (your behaviors, feelings, thoughts, attitudes) or themes you notice in your relationships.

5. Describe any similar interpersonal patterns (your behaviors, feelings, thoughts, attitudes) that you've observed between your nuclear family and your romantic relationships.

6. What do you feel you need to work on to improve your interpersonal relationships?

7. Identify one thing you are willing to practice to improve your relationships.

Exploring Interpersonal Problems and Social Functioning

The relationships of people with an insecure style of attachment who come from family systems that are unsupportive with a high level of conflict suffer (Tasca 2019). Individuals that have these challenges need to learn ways to deal with interpersonal and social situations. For example, they may not realize that they have unrealistic expectations of their partner, or are highly distressed during life transitions, have social sensitivities, or are not aware of their emotional triggers that elicit their insecure activating coping strategies (highly reactive, controlling).

Therefore, it is important for them to learn what their emotional triggers are and how to effectively cope through stressful events. This is essential because individuals with insecure attachment can be highly distressed, and their propensity to utilize activating and deactivating coping strategies will ultimately sabotage their relationships. This cycle will continue until individuals have awareness about themselves, their tendencies, their reactions, and choose to cope with the intensity of their emotions in a more effective way. This is the focus of the next chapter, foundational skill #7 *Coping with Emotional Triggers and Building Resilience*.

Bibliography

Abbate-Daga, G. et al. (2010). Attachment insecurity, personality, and body dissatisfaction in eating disorders. *The Journal of Nervous and Mental Disease*, *198*(7), 520–524. https://doi.org/10.1097/NMD.0b013e3181e4c6f7.

Ambwani, S., Roche, M. J., Minnick, A. M., & Pincus, A. L. (2015). Negative affect, interpersonal perception, and binge eating behavior: An experience sampling study. *International Journal of Eating Disorders*, *48*(6), 715–726. DOI: 10.1002/eat.22410.

Bosmans, G., & Borelli, J. L. (2022). Attachment and the Development of Psychopathology: Introduction to the Special Issue. *Brain Sciences*, *12*(2), 174. https://doi.org/10.3390/brainsci12020174.

Cassidy, J., Jones, J. D., & Shaver, P. R. (2013). Contributions of attachment theory and research: a framework for future research, translation, and policy. *Development and Psychopathology*, *25*(4 Pt 2), 1415–1434. https://doi.org/10.1017/S0954579413000692.

Cortés-García, L., Takkouche, B., Seoane, G., & Senra, C. (2019). Mediators linking insecure attachment to eating symptoms: A systematic review and meta-analysis. *PLoS ONE*, *14*(3), Article e0213099. https://doi.org/10.1371/journal.pone.0213099.

De Groot, J., & Rodin, G. (1998). Coming alive: the psychotherapeutic treatment of patients with eating disorders. *Canadian Journal of Psychiatry*, *43*(4), 359–60. DOI: 10.1177/070674379804300403.

Erriu, M., Cimino, S., & Cerniglia, L. (2020). The Role of Family Relationships in Eating Disorders in Adolescents: A Narrative Review. *Behavioral Sciences (Basel, Switzerland)*, *10*(4), 71. https://doi.org/10.3390/bs10040071.

Gagliardi, M. (2021). How Our Caregivers Shape Who We Are: The Seven Dimensions of Attachment at the Core of Personality. *Frontiers in Psychology*, *12*, 657628. https://doi.org/10.3389/fpsyg.2021.657628.

Gander, M., Sevecke, K., & Buchheim, A. (2015). Eating disorders in adolescence: attachment issues from a developmental perspective. *Frontiers in Psychology*, *6*, 1136. https://doi.org/10.3389/fpsyg.2015.01136.

Girme, Y. U. et al. (2018). The ebbs and flows of attachment: Within-person variation in attachment undermine secure individuals' relationship wellbeing across time. *Journal of Personality and Social Psychology*, *114*(3), 397–421. https://doi.org/10.1037/pspi0000115.

Girme, Y. U. et al. (2021). Infants' attachment insecurity predicts attachment-relevant emotion regulation strategies in adulthood. *Emotion (Washington, D.C.)*, *21*(2), 260–272. https://doi.org/10.1037/emo0000721.

Ivanova, I. V., Tasca, G. A., Proulx, G., & Bissada, H. (2017). Contribution of Interpersonal Problems to Eating Disorder Psychopathology via Negative Affect in Treatment-seeking Men and Women: Testing the Validity of the Interpersonal Model in an Understudied Population. *Clin Psychol Psychother*,[Q9] *24*(4), 952–964. DOI: 10.1002/cpp.2060.

Kaurin, A., Pilkonis, P. A., & Wright, A. G. C. (2022). Attachment manifestations in daily interpersonal interactions. *Affective Science*. Advance online publication. https://doi.org/10.1007/s42761-022-00117-6.

Keating, L., Tasca, G. A., & Hill, R. (2013). Structural relationships among attachment insecurity, alexithymia, and body esteem in women with eating disorders. *Eating Behaviors*, *14*(3), 366–373. https://doi.org/10.1016/j.eatbeh.2013.06.013.

Kirby, J. S. et al. (2015). Couple-Based Interventions for Adults with Eating Disorders. *Eating Disorders*, *23*(4), 356–365. https://doi.org/10.1080/10640266.2015.1044349.

Kuipers, G. S., den Hollander, S., van der Ark, L. A., & Bekker, M. H. J. (2017). Recovery from eating disorder 1 year after start of treatment is related to better mentalization and strong reduction of sensitivity to others. *Eating and Weight Disorders*, *22*(3), 535–547. Advance online publication. https://doi.org/10.1007/s40519-017-0405-x .

Lenzo, V. et al. (2021). The Interplay of Attachment Styles and Defense Mechanisms on Eating Disorders Risk: Cross-Sectional Observation in the Community Population. *Clinical Neuropsychiatry*, *18*(6), 296–303. DOI: 10.36131/cnfioritieditore20210603.

Lev Arey, D., Sagi, A. & Blatt, A. (2023). The relationship between exercise addiction, eating disorders, and insecure attachment styles among recreational exercisers. *Journal of Eating Disorders, 11,* 131. https://doi.org/10.1186/s40337-023-00855-3.

Mason, T. B. et al.(2016). The role of interpersonal personality traits and reassurance seeking in eating disorder symptoms and depressive symptoms among women with bulimia nervosa. *Comprehensive Psychiatry, 68,* 165–171. https://doi.org/10.1016/j.comppsych.2016.04.013.

Mason, T. B. et al.(2022). A systematic review of maladaptive interpersonal behaviors and eating disorder psychopathology. *Eating Behaviors, 45,* 101601. https://doi.org/10.1016/j.eatbeh.2022.101601.

Monteleone, A. M. et al. (2019). The association between childhood maltreatment and eating disorder psychopathology: A mixed-model investigation. *European Psychiatry, 61,* 111–118. DOI: 10.1016/j.eurpsy.2019.08.002.

Monteleone, A. M. et al.(2020). Parental bonding, childhood maltreatment and eating disorder psychopathology: an investigation of their interactions. *Eating and Weight Disorders: EWD, 25*(3), 577–589. https://doi.org/10.1007/s40519-019-00649-0.

Monteleone, A. M. et al. (2022). The connection between childhood maltreatment and eating disorder psychopathology: a network analysis study in people with bulimia nervosa and with binge eating disorder. *Eating and weight disorders: EWD, 27*(1), 253–261. https://doi.org/10.1007/s40519-021-01169-6.

Tasca, G. A. (2019). Attachment and eating disorders: A research update. *Current Opinion in Psychology, 25,* 59–64. https://doi.org/10.1016/j.copsyc.2018.03.003.

Troisi, A., Massaroni, P., & Cuzzolaro, M. (2005). Early separation anxiety and adult attachment style in women with eating disorders. *British Journal of Clinical Psychology, 44*(Pt 1), 89–97.

Troisi, A. et al. (2006). Body Dissatisfaction in Women With Eating Disorders: Relationship to Early Separation Anxiety and Insecure Attachment. *Psychosomatic Medicine, 68,* 449–453. 10.1097/01.psy.0000204923.09390.5b.

Foundational Skill #7

Coping with Emotional Triggers and Building Resilience

The ability to emotionally regulate is imperative for long term recovery from an eating disorder. People who struggle with eating often struggle with identifying, describing, and tolerating their emotions (Foye et al. 2017). Therefore, learning to recognize emotional triggers, identifying effective coping strategies, practicing emotional tolerance, and eventually building emotional resilience are essential for lasting recovery (Dingemans et al. 2017). Overall, emotion regulation does not differ across eating disorders—problems in regulating emotions are characteristic of eating pathology (Prefit et al. 2019).

In this chapter, your client will build on previous foundational skills and use them in conjunction with foundational skill *#7 Coping with Emotional Triggers and Building Resilience*. With practice, these skills will develop naturally and will be integrated in your client's daily life.

Your client will learn, identify, and practice skills by using worksheets and exercises. This chapter covers the following:

- Identifying factors that cause vulnerability to emotion dysregulation.
- Understanding the window of tolerance.
- Recognizing the function of eating disorder behaviors in coping with emotions.
- Identifying emotional triggers.
- Understanding emotional firing order.
- Developing protectors for emotional resilience.

Vulnerability to Emotion Dysregulation

Many factors can contribute to the vulnerability of emotional dysregulation. Here are some examples that may contribute to your client's challenges in regulating their emotions.

Sensitivity and Temperament

Some individuals are naturally more emotionally sensitive and experience feelings more intensely and may have endured negative criticism such as, "You're so sensitive" or "It was just a joke— what's wrong with you?" These comments results in individuals denying and suppressing their emotions out of fear of being negatively judged. Further, self-directed behaviors such as blame and criticism contribute to emotional dysregulation (Monell et al. 2020).

> *Rachel: "My dad always questioned why I felt a certain way. His facial expressions towards me made me feel like I was weird or something."*

DOI: 10.4324/9781032651408-14

Family

Our clients learned from a young age that there are acceptable and unacceptable emotions. Expressing undesirable emotions such as anger could leave them susceptible to rejection. Their early experiences in family could be overwhelming, lacking emotional expression, or emotionally explosive and volatile.

> Rachel: "If I was sad or angry I was considered a drama queen—something was wrong with me because it didn't bother anyone else in the family."

Poor Emotional Development and Lack of Skills

Identifying, describing, and recognizing their emotions are often difficult. Overwhelming emotions such as anger, sadness, worry, loneliness, depression, disgust, frustration, and guilt feel intolerable. They may believe that their emotions are a sign of weakness and fear losing control when engulfed with feelings.

> Rachel: "I don't even know what I feel sometimes. I just can't explain it but I all I know is I just want to eat. I just don't know what to do so I just try not to feel anything. I know something is wrong because I can't stop eating."

Trauma Response

Some individuals may be dealing with unresolved trauma and their emotions and discomfort can feel unsafe in their body. Noticeable changes in the way they feel can trigger a past trauma and elicit feelings of helplessness. In contrast, they may also feel completely disconnected and dissociated with no awareness of their emotions.

> Rachel: "I get out of control calling my boyfriend because I go to a place where I panic. I can't focus until he answers the phone and I feel so desperate, like I'm dying."

Window of Tolerance

Building emotional resilience requires individuals to develop the ability to connect to their physical body—not disconnect it from it. However, this step can be the most challenging for them. Their past inclination of engaging in maladaptive numbing behaviors to disconnect have been their way of coping. Therefore, it is important that individuals practice skills found in Chapter 3, foundational skill #1 *Establishing a Mind-Body Connection*. This skill is used together with identifying emotional triggers and in learning to build emotional resilience.

Dr. Daniel Siegel introduced the "window of tolerance" in his book, *The Developing Mind* (Siegel 2012). The "window of tolerance" is a metaphor used to help clients recognize their range of experience with emotional intensity. This is important because everyone has a different tolerance level of emotional discomfort. Therefore, clients need to learn to recognize and identify their limits and when they are outside of their emotional window. Having this information will help them practice strategies to stay in—and the ability to return to—their calm space.

The "window of tolerance" model describes every window as having an upper and a lower boundary. The hyper-arousal state (upper boundary zone), for example, is recognized as irritability, severe anxiety, hypervigilance, aggression, difficulty concentrating, or agitation. In contrast, individuals that are in a hypo-arousal state (lower boundary zone), for example, may experience disconnection, withdrawal, fatigue, feelings of hopelessness, brain fog, and feelings of emptiness. When your clients are in these zones their ability to function effectively, stay present and focused is disrupted. In comparison, when individuals are in the window of tolerance, they are calm, alert, focused, and can function effectively.

Identifying and recognizing body sensations and emotions gives your clients the ability to utilize strategies to return to their calm space when they are outside of their window. They will practice this in the next exercise.

CLIENT EXERCISE: AWARENESS OF INTENSITY OF EMOTIONS

Bringing greater awareness to your emotions—and their level of intensity—is an important part of managing your feelings well. Think of it as the first tool you'll need to in your coping toolbox.

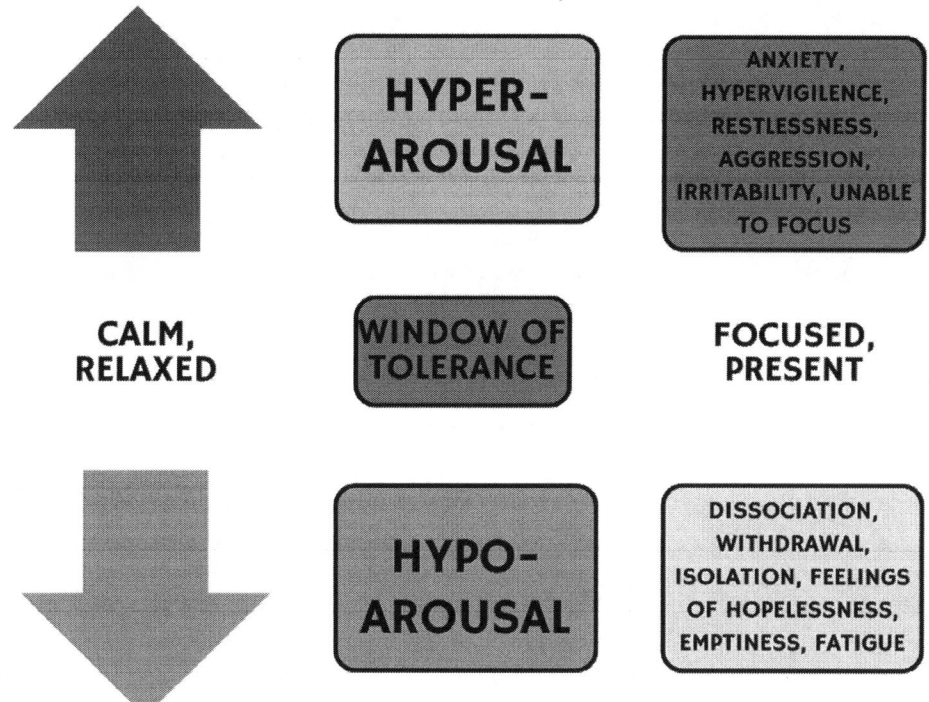

Figure 9.1 Window of Tolerance

Objective: To better acquaint yourself with your emotions for effective emotion regulation.

Directions: Look at the three intensity of emotion zones in the diagram. Then answer the questions by describing what you experience when you are in each of the zones.

1. Describe what you experience when you are in the hyper-arousal zone? What keeps you there?

2. Describe what you experience when you are in the "window of tolerance?" What keeps you there?

3. Describe what you experience when you are in the hypo-arousal zone? What keeps you there?

Because intense emotions can feel debilitating, when individuals do not have the capacity to utilize skills in this activated state, mental models can be extremely helpful for dealing with the unknown. This helps individuals feel more in control of their feelings and makes ambiguous feelings less intense. Using a mental model as a reference gives your client a way to identify the strategies to help them return to their window of tolerance. For example, after completing the previous worksheet, Rachel began to gain clarity around the boundaries of her tolerance:

Rachel: "I know I'm starting to leave my window of calmness when my mind starts to wander. I'm no longer focused and starting to think about why my boyfriend hasn't returned my call. This is my sign that something is wrong and I need to take a walk or call a friend. My mind will start thinking about bad things and before I know it, I am in a full-blown panic attack."

Rachel recognizes that when her mind wanders it is an indicator that her body is leaving her calm, relaxed state. Because Rachel has been practicing these skills, she recognizes that her distress can spiral out of control quickly. This is the point where her ability to choose an adaptive skill is high. However, when her distress increases, her flexibility and openness in trying a newer alternative skill decrease. It will be more difficult for her to return to a regulated state—resulting in using maladaptive strategies that she knows is effective.

The Function of Eating Disorder Behaviors in Coping with Emotions

Maladaptive behaviors can be tough to eliminate because not only are they functional, they are highly effective. Eating disorder behaviors help clients, numb, distract, suppress, and cope through negative effects and emotional discomfort (Ortiz et al. 2022). Your clients try to regulate their emotions by re-directing them towards their bodies (Henderson et al. 2019) Let's take a look at some examples of how these behaviors function when used to regulate negative emotions.

- Emotional eating/binging: *"When I'm eating, I tune everything out. At first, I'm excited to eat. And then by the end of it, I'm not thinking about anything except how physically full and uncomfortable I feel. Then I'm like why did I do that?"* (Self-soothing and distraction)
- Restricting food: *"When there are hard emotions, I immediately feel like I have a stomachache. I feel nauseated and feel so full. I don't want to eat. Other times, I may just not want to feel anymore and I just want to disconnect from feeling anything."* (Numbing, controlling, disconnecting)
- Purging (self-induced vomiting, laxative use): *"It feels so gross in my body. I need to get rid of whatever I'm feeling. I can feel dirty or messy and or just bad. I need to get rid of the grossness in my body".* (Controlling, and releasing)
- Compulsive over-exercising: *"When I run for miles, it helps me not to think or feel anything."* (Distraction, disconnecting, releasing)
- Diet pills or fasting: *"It just helps me to feel like I'm doing something to control my weight and I can feel less anxious."* (Controlling, disconnecting)
- Chew spitting: *"I can get rid of whatever I'm not okay with I eat it, but I feel better because I can also spit it out."* (Controlling, self-soothing)
- Rumination: *"I bring up the food and chew again and swallow. I don't even know when I'm doing it anymore. I know it sounds gross, but it's calming me and soothes me."* (Calming, self-soothing)
- Body checking: *"When things feel really uncomfortable, like when I have doubt about something, rubbing my collar bone, or my hip bone lets me know I'm okay."* (Self-soothing, controlling, calming.)
- The eating disorder voice: *"Sometimes just paying attention to the voice helps me calm all other thoughts. Just tuning into the voice can help me feel better because it can sound supportive and helps distracts me from what's going on, like it says, at least you can diet, or just don't eat, you'll feel better. I feel like I'm not alone and it's a supportive friend, but other times it can get me back on track by yelling at me. The voice says, 'stop being so sensitive and get over it.'"* (Soothing, calming, empowering)

It is helpful for your client to explore what they are feeling and increase their awareness about how they've been coping through tough emotions.

CLIENT WORKSHEET: IDENTIFYING EATING DISORDER COPING BEHAVIORS

What do you tend to do when things get hard? Do you engage in eating disorder behaviors to cope? If so, you might wind up feeling guilty or angry afterwards, knowing that your actions weren't the best choice. And then to stop feeling guilty or angry, you might use another eating disorder behavior to numb your feelings. But that's a vicious cycle! However, you can stop this habit by learning to use proactive behaviors before you're outside of your window of tolerance.

Objective: Gain awareness about unhelpful cycle-maintaining coping strategies and their consequences, along with helpful cycle-ending strategies that you can use instead.

Directions: Complete the questions below and discuss with your therapist.

What unhelpful eating disorder behavior do you use to deal with your intense emotions?	How does this behavior add to or exacerbate your negative emotions?	What are the results of using this behavior? How does it affect the way you feel about yourself and your relationships with others?
What helpful behaviors have you used in the past to deal with intense emotions? Or what helpful behaviors would you want to try when a negative feeling creeps up?	How does (or would) this helpful behavior help you with your negative emotions?	What are the results of using a helpful behavior? How does (or would) it affect the way you feel about yourself and your relationships with others?

Emotional Triggers

Most clients who struggle with eating experience frequent and intense mood fluctuations known as *affective lability*. People with high lability experience rapid fluctuations in emotions—and tend to engage in maladaptive behaviors for immediate relief. Studies have shown that there is a positive connection between people who struggle with disordered eating and affective lability (Ortiz et al. 2022).

Emotional triggers can derail recovery if individuals do not have the skills to effectively deal with the stimulus. Most of the time, emotional triggers are unexpected and individuals are not prepared for the emotional intensity in that moment. People who struggle with food also tend to have difficulty with flexibility, making things even more challenging. Therefore, they try to mitigate these issues by avoiding situations that can provoke uncomfortable feelings. However, this adds to their problems by increasing difficulty in psychosocial functioning. Psychosocial functioning will be discussed in the next chapter, foundational skill #8 *Using My Authentic Voice*. The following are common emotional triggers for people struggling with disordered eating.

Fear and Disgust

When individuals experience fear, it is usually manifested in their eating disorder. It can be expressed as fear of weight gain, losing control of eating, and judgments about their body and appearance. Examples of underlying issues of fear are fear of rejection, not being accepted, not being lovable, not being enough, or not feeling worthy. These feelings can trigger a quick spiral usually brought on by conflict in their interpersonal relationships.

When our clients experience disgust, it is also usually manifested in their eating disorder by eating, viewing themselves in the mirror, or their judgements about their body image. This emotion is triggered by social vulnerability and challenging social situations.

Shame

Shame is one of the most painful emotions. Individuals who struggle with emotion regulation often identify anger, sadness, and guilt as the most difficult—and often don't realize that it's shame they are experiencing. When they feel this pain, they want to escape, disappear, or to punish themselves because they see themselves in the most harsh, critical way. They feel as though something is inherently wrong with them—feeling "small," inferior, helpless, powerless, and exposed. This can bring on shame from earlier memories, intensifying the body discomfort—and causing them to react by escaping their feelings.

Let's take a look at how shame affects your client.

Review Rachel's completed example to help your client complete the worksheet.

RACHEL'S WORKSHEET: THE TRIGGER OF SHAME

---

1. How do you know you are experiencing shame? How does shame affect your thoughts?
   (Examples: There's something weird about me. Everyone thinks I'm stupid. I just want to disappear.)

   I repeat over and over again how stupid I am. "I am so stupid" is always the thought. I always tell myself how stupid I am for thinking someone could love me.

2. What do you notice in your body (physical sensations)?
   (Examples: Hard to breathe, constriction, heat and discomfort in chest.)

   I have this icky feeling, and like my body is vibrating hot energy. I can't breathe, and I feel this gross feeling in my body that makes me want to disappear.

3. What do you notice in your behaviors?
   (Examples: Shrink down, no eye contact with anyone, shoulders slouch and face down.)

   I can't look at anyone and I feel like I'm completely exposed, like everyone sees how bad I am. I'm sure I'm making weird facial expressions because in that moment, I don't even know how to act. I can't smile nor

---

do I want to, but I try to so that people don't know that I'm affected but then it everyone notices, because my facial expression just looks weird.

4. What's the story behind shame that comes to mind for you?
    (Example: Usually something that feels like an absolute: like always or never.)

    The story usually goes, "this is what you get for being stupid", or "Why the heck do you think things will work out for you, you aren't special." "Why are you so stupid?"

5. How do you feel shame is helpful or unhelpful?

    It's helpful because I try to avoid doing things that will bring shame. But unhelpful because I have a tendency to avoid everything in fear that it will bring shame to me.

6. How do you feel shame affects your interpersonal relationships?

    I give and do everything for everyone else and they end up taking advantage of me because I feel so much shame for asking for what I need. I don't have needs but then I get angry that I'm not getting my needs met, and it goes in a cycle. I haven't had any real healthy relationships because of it.

7. How do you feel shame affects you socially?

    I make myself as small as possible. I try to avoid it if possible or I tend to not bring attention on to me.

8. Imagine if you did not experience shame, what do you feel you could do? What has the fear of experiencing shame been holding you back from?

    One of my biggest fears is failure. I feel a lot of shame around failing. If I didn't feel shame, I would take risks, put myself out there and be seen. Shame is holding me back from everything. It is holding me back from life.

CLIENT WORKSHEET: THE TRIGGER OF SHAME

Can you remember the last time you experienced shame? What did it feel like? What did you do? Shame is experienced as a deeply painful emotional experience. Like all other emotions shame is loaded with information and can motivate a change in behavior. However, while shame can motivate you to conform to what might be most socially acceptable, it can also cause reactions that are not helpful. Let's explore how you have experienced shame and how it affects you.

Objective: Create awareness about shame and how it affects our ability to function.
Directions: Complete the following questions and discuss with your therapist.

1. How do you know you are experiencing shame? How does shame affect your thoughts?

    (Examples: There's something weird about me. Everyone thinks I'm stupid. I just want to disappear.)

2. What do you notice in your body (physical sensations)?

    (Examples: Hard to breathe, constriction, heat and discomfort in chest.)

3. What do you notice in your behaviors?

    (Examples: Shrink down, no eye contact with anyone, shoulders slouch and face down.)

4. What's the story behind shame that comes to mind for you?

    (Example: Usually something that feels like an absolute: like always or never.)

5. How do you feel shame is helpful or unhelpful?

6. How do you feel shame affects your interpersonal relationships?

7. How do you feel shame affects you socially?

8. Imagine if you did not experience shame, what do you feel you could do? What has the fear of experiencing shame been holding you back from?

Interpersonal Relationships

Interactions with people can be emotionally triggering for individuals struggling with eating disorders.

Often, they don't know how to respond or cope with triggering behaviors by others. (Teaching your clients how to respond and communicate with others will be addressed in the next chapter, foundational skill #8 *Using My Authentic Voice.*) They tend to deal with it by laughing it off, ignoring or even agreeing with the others' comments but when they are alone they replay the activating interactions in their head. They obsess on parts that bother them the most, the parts that elicit negative feelings, thoughts, and images.

These interpersonal triggers can remind your clients of past experiences. It can also be emotionally disturbing because the person may be a reminder of another with negative associations. This can bring up intense emotions since your client may not be aware what caused the stimulus.

Examples of how Rachel was affected by others in her previous sessions.

"I asked my boyfriend how I looked, and he said, 'fine' in that tone. The tone that doesn't mean fine."

Rachel was bothered by the tone of her boyfriend's response. The tone reminded Rachel of the tone her mother used when she was upset. It is a trigger because she always felt that she was never "good enough" in her mother's eyes.

"I don't like seeing my family. My aunt always makes comments about my weight. It's so triggering for me. The last time I saw her, she said, 'Your dress looks a little tight, are you okay?'"

Rachel's aunt's words activated Rachel's own negative judgments, thoughts, and dissatisfaction about her body image.

"I ran into my coach from high school at the mall. He looked me up and down and made a face like he was disgusted, and then he walked away without acknowledging me."

Rachel created a story in her mind and projected her own feelings of disgust and thinking on to her coach.

"I was in line at the post office, and my neighbor's little girl looked at me—she pointed at me, and said, 'She's fat, mom.'"

Rachel's own negative beliefs and judgments about herself make the little girl's comments more difficult to hear. Rachel's fear is being judged and found unlovable by others. The little girl's words triggered Rachel's fears and confirmed that the whole world sees her this way.

Let's look at some practice exercises in creating awareness around their interpersonal triggers.

CLIENT WORKSHEET: UNCOVERING INTERPERSONAL TRIGGERS

Have you ever been bothered by someone but couldn't quite pinpoint what it is about them or what they are doing that is bothering you? Or maybe you know exactly what the other person said that bothers you but are having trouble understanding why you can't stop thinking about it and why it's affecting you.

Let's practice increasing your awareness about what is really bothering you in order to work through it.

Practice asking yourself these questions when you feel triggered by an interaction with someone.

Identify the behavior of the other person that was triggering for you.	What bothered you <u>most</u> about their behavior?	Does this person's behavior remind you of anyone? If so, who? How?	What does the feeling you are experiencing remind you of?	Could this situation remind you of another situation? If so, what?

Identify the behavior of the other person that was triggering for you.	What bothered you most about their behavior?	Does this person's behavior remind you of anyone? If so, who? How?	What does the feeling you are experiencing remind you of?	Could this situation remind you of another situation? If so, what?

Social Anxiety

People who struggle with eating disorders also struggle with *cognitive inflexibility*. This is a lack of awareness of options when unexpected conditions arise. They are also unwilling to adapt in these situations (Arlt et al. 2016) and have great difficulty engaging in social activities and with psychosocial functioning.

Their social anxiety is increased because they aren't confident that they would be able to handle various situations. For example, they may fear others' negative judgments, social situations, or unexpected and unplanned circumstances around food, or experience anxiety with just the thought of being seen by others.

They avoid situations where their bodies may be exposed such as beach events, pool parties, and outdoor activities. Further, they usually decline events that are centered around food, such as buffets or where others will notice their eating behaviors or choices of food.

> *Rachel: "I don't like going out with groups. What if people order food that I don't eat? I will feel so anxious and nervous sitting there and I feel like I want to disappear."*

Rachel would rather avoid social situations altogether rather than to have to experience the discomfort of having to communicate what she would like to order.

Let's take a look at how your client can practice flexibility in their thinking when dealing with social situations.

CLIENT EXERCISE: PRACTICE FLEXIBILITY

Have you ever been in a situation and wished you had dealt with it differently? Maybe you were caught off guard and so you had no idea what to do. Or maybe you believed there was only one way to deal with the situation, and so you acted on it. In this exercise, let's practice looking at a difficult situation in various ways.

Objective: Increase flexibility of perception of challenging situations.
Directions: Complete the questions and discuss with your therapist.

1. Describe a difficult social situation.

2. What did you do in the situation? What was the outcome of the situation?

3. If you didn't have to experience any consequences, insecurities, or anxieties about this situation, what would you have done instead?

4. What do you think the outcome would have been if you did that (with no experience of any consequences, insecurities, or anxieties)?

5. How do you feel the person you admire most would have handled that situation?

6. How do you feel the person you have most challenges with would have handled that situation?

7. How would you handle a situation like that in the future?

Loneliness

Loneliness is another emotional trigger for individuals who struggle with eating and they often use food as a way to comfort and soothe feelings of loneliness. This is exasperated by their issues with interpersonal relationships and struggles with social anxiety. They experience loneliness because of a lack of quality relationships and meaningful connections. This can be taxing on any existing relationship that they may have due to their demands on their partners. They can feel overwhelmed and drained by the responsibility of filling the void for their loneliness, causing more interpersonal turmoil. It is important that those who have difficulty with loneliness practice coping through feelings, develop a social support system, and increase social functioning (Momeñe et al. 2022).

Studies have shown that there is a link between secure attachment and oxytocin (Buchheim et al. 2009) and that it plays a central role in interpersonal relationships, especially through prosocial behaviors such as helping a friend, mentoring a child, doing community service, or helping the elderly with chores. These relationships boost oxytocin (Vitale & Smith 2022). Researchers found that gratitude is closely linked to oxytocin (Algoe et al. 2017). It has been shown that oxytocin is increased in interpersonal relationships and that intentional acts and practicing gratitude can decrease subjective feelings of loneliness. Gratitude is a reminder that they have people that they are connected to—helping them feel more optimistic and satisfied in general.

In the next exercise, your client will practice acknowledging gratitude for what they have in their life.

CLIENT EXERCISE: GRATITUDE

Some days can be hard, and we may have a tendency to focus only on the negative aspects of our life. Have you ever stopped to think about all the things that have been going well in your life? Let's take a moment to acknowledge people, situations, and things in your life that you appreciate.

Objective: Practice gratitude to increase *oxytocin*, the feel-good hormone, and to feel more optimistic and uplift mood.
Directions: Complete gratitude list daily before bed or at the start of the day.

Write down five things you are grateful for:

1.

2.

3.

4.

5.

Intuition

Your clients may experience intuition—the physical sensation of "knowing"—as intensely uncomfortable in their body. They can also misinterpret these sensations for other body cues such as hunger, fullness, or it may even bring up unresolved past trauma. For example:

Rachel: "I have awful sensations in the pit of my stomach when I know something is wrong. I felt it as a kid and I still feel it as an adult. I hate that feeling. I know when someone is lying or when someone has bad news and are hiding it. It feels so bad I want to throw up. Only throwing up relieves that feeling for me."

I will never forget the first time I felt the sensation. My mom dropped me off at my grandma's house when I was five. I just knew that she was lying and that she wouldn't be right back like she said she was. I was right. She came back weeks later to pick me up. I just don't understand why she would lie to me, and I felt sick that whole time she was gone. Whenever I have the feeling in my gut, I do everything I can to not feel it, but then it gets so strong like I have to throw up."

Like Rachel, many have challenges with emotion regulation when they have a strong physical sensation that something is wrong. Extreme anxiety often accompanies the discomfort they are feeling in the pit of their stomach. Therefore, it is common for individuals to mistake intuition for anxiety or the other way around. In the next exercise, your clients will explore the difference between experiencing intuition and anxiety.

Therapist Tips:

It is common for your clients to struggle with recognizing their intuition.

- *Intuition can be learned by observing body cues, thoughts, and feelings.*
- *They can observe and reflect and wait for situations to naturally unfold to check whether they were right about their intuition,*
- *Practicing will give them more information for future situations.*

CLIENT EXERCISE: INTUITION VERSUS ANXIETY

Have you ever had a strange feeling that something is wrong but dismissed it as anxiety? Have you ever considered that that feeling may actually have been your intuition? Or have you ever experienced extreme anxiety and mistaken it for intuition? Well, if you've experienced this, you know how uncomfortable this can be. Let's learn more about the differences you experience with intuition and anxiety.

Merriam-Webster defines *intuition* as:

1. immediate apprehension or cognition without reasoning or inferring.
2. knowledge or conviction gained by intuition.
3. the power or faculty of gaining direct knowledge or cognition without evident rational thought and inference.

Anxiety is defined as:

1. apprehensive uneasiness or nervousness usually over an impending or anticipated ill.
2. mentally distressing concern or interest.
3. a strong desire sometimes mixed with doubt, fear, or uneasiness.

Objective: Differentiate between intuition and anxiety, as well as hunger and fullness.
Directions: Using markers, pens, or crayons complete the following in Figure 9.2:

1. Draw (in the figure), where you feel your intuition.
2. Write (in the figure) the physical sensations you experience as intuition.
3. Draw (in the figure), where you feel anxiety.
4. Write (in the figure) the physical sensations you experience as anxiety.
5. Draw (in the figure) where you feel your hunger/fullness.
6. Write (in the figure) the physical sensations you experience as hunger/fullness.
7. Answer reflection questions.

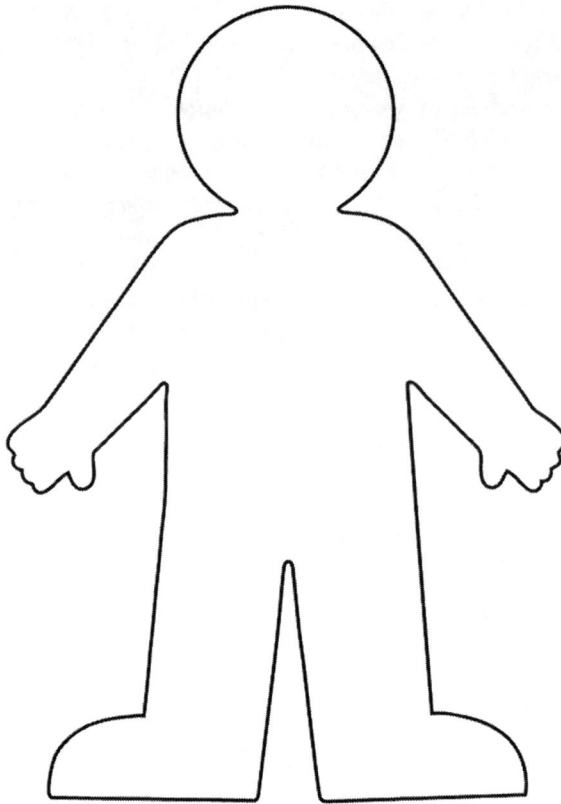

Figure 9.2 Outline of Body.

Reflection questions

1. Describe a time when you were right about your intuition. What did you feel in your body? What were your thoughts and feelings?

2. Describe a time when you were right about your anxiety. What did you feel in your body? What were your thoughts and feelings?

3. Describe a time when you were right about your hunger cues. What did you feel in your body? What were your thoughts and feelings?

4. What helped you to differentiate the three experiences?

Recognizing the Firing Order of Triggers

Now that your client can practice integrating their physical sensations with their emotional feelings and thoughts, let's take a look at what bothers your client most. Studies show that emotional intelligence plays a key role in reducing symptomatology of eating disorders resulting in increased self-esteem and reduced anxiety symptoms (Peláez-Fernández et al. 2022). Individuals react differently when they become emotionally dysregulated. For some, the imagery that goes with the activating event bothers them most. This initiates their emotional process of spiraling out of control. However, for others it could be their thoughts or their physical sensations that sparks their emotional dysregulation.

When individuals are able to recognize their emotional firing order, they are able to understand what is happening (Meneguzzo et al. 2019). They will feel more grounded and more regulated. The unexpected and intense nature of emotions feel overwhelming. They struggle with the intensity of the emotion hitting them all at once because it feels "out of control"—which is another trigger that adds fuel to the fire.

> *Rachel: "When I get triggered and feel like someone is going to leave me, I feel immediately helpless, and like I am going to die. I feel like a baby. When this happens, I realize, the first thing that sparks the thought (He's leaving me.). Then I feel like I can't breathe, so the physical sensations start. My heart pounds fast. The physical sensations make me feel so scared. It's definitely the sensations that bother me the most. Then the emotions and lastly the imagery. I feel like I can't even imagine anything at the moment because my mind is black and all I just feel is pure ickiness in my body, like I'm dying. It's intense."*

Rachel is reacting to her boyfriend leaving the relationship and doesn't have the communication skills to express how she feels. Therefore, the relationship ends with her boyfriend leaving. Her emotional firing order in this situation is:

> *Cognition (thoughts)—physical sensations—emotions—imagery*

When individuals are able to recognize their firing order in each situation, they are less affected by the unpredictability and can choose a skill relevant to the intensity of their firing order.

Also, note that their firing order can be different depending on the situation. It would be highly effective for your client to keep this in mind and to practice this skill daily with less intense situations. This will help your client create consciousness which is important for eating disorder recovery (Leppanen et al. 2022).

Let's try this with your client.

CLIENT EXERCISE: TRACKING THE FIRING ORDER OF EMOTIONAL TRIGGERS

Emotional triggers can be intense and challenging—especially because they are unexpected. This can be extremely overwhelming because you may be experiencing several emotions all at once. In this exercise, we break down what happens when the trigger is initiated. Let's take a look at you firing order—how the trigger affects you—and what bothers you most in the process. What happens when an emotional trigger occurs? What do you notice occurs first? The self-regulation awareness tool depicts what happens when you are activated by an emotional trigger. Everyone is unique in the order of this process.

Objective: Create awareness by using the Self-Regulation Awareness Tool to discover your firing order.
Directions: Review Figure 9.3. Next, read Rachel's completed worksheet to give you a sense of one of many ways to answer the questions. Then answer the questions for yourself and discuss with your therapist.

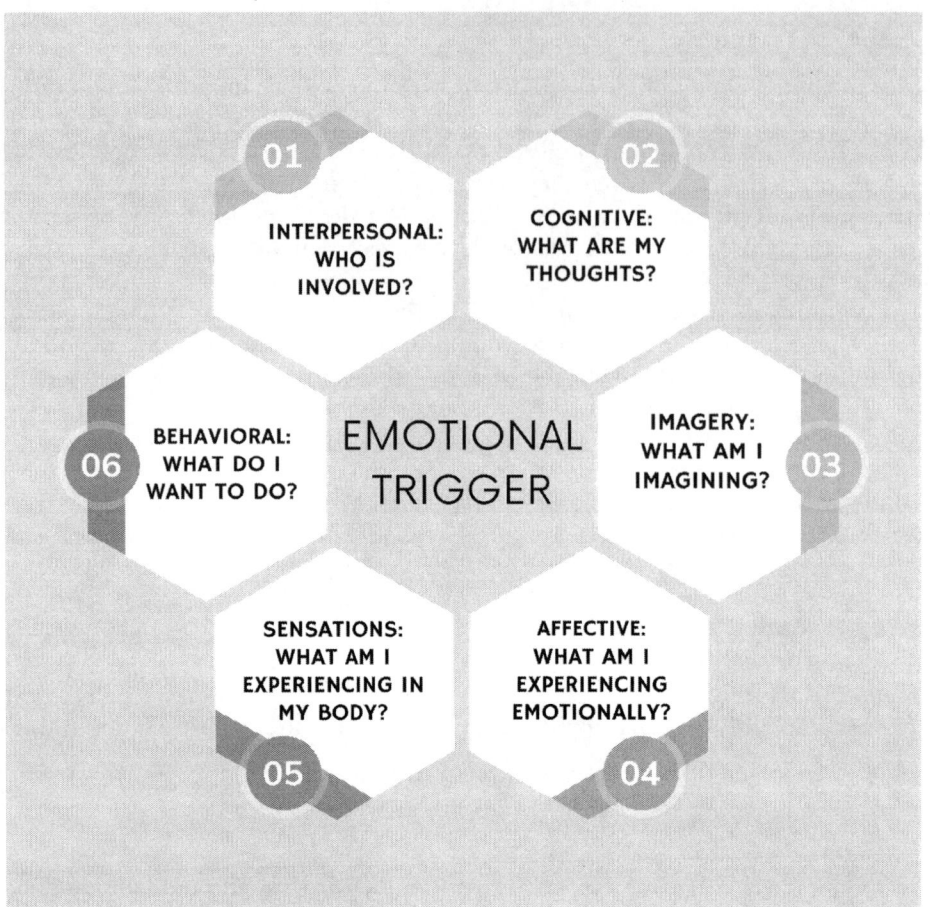

Figure 9.3 Self-Regulation Awareness Tool

RACHEL'S WORKSHEET

1. Identify (describe) an emotional trigger or a challenging situation.

    I was going through my boyfriend's phone, and I saw a photo of another woman.

2. What was the interaction with the other person?

    I didn't tell him I saw it because I'm not supposed to be going through his things.

3. How did you behave in the situation?

    I shut down, cried. I paced a lot. I didn't know what to do.

4. What are your thoughts about the trigger or situation?

    My thoughts were really confused. I had a lot of questions like, is he cheating? Who is this person? How long has it been going on? Is it serious? How could he do that?

5. What did you sense in your body (physical sensations)?

    My heart is beating fast. I couldn't breathe. I felt frozen. I felt dizzy. I felt like I wanted to throw up. I needed to lay down and cry at the same time. But I was too much in shock to cry, right away.

6. What emotions did you experience?

Betrayal, grief, anger, sadness.

7. What did you imagine?

I imagined him cheating on me and talking to on the phone with this person. I imagined the worst.

8. Indicate the firing order of the processes and what you notice first to the last (use the diagram).

I notice I imagine the worst, then my I feel all the discomfort in my body, then my emotions, then my thoughts. I usually have no idea what to do or how to go about dealing with it with the other person. I also pace while I'm going through all of it. I think I'm frozen so the interpersonal interaction is last. I need time to calm down before I can talk about it. I tend to isolate first.

9. Put the processes in order from which they bother you the most to the least?

This is the same order as what I notice happening first.

10. What does this process tell you about yourself?

It tells me that things are always really bad for me because I always go to the worst-case scenario. I will always imagine the worst, so it will always be really bad for me. Everything happens afterwards is because of the worst story in my mind, even if it may not be true.

11. What do you need?

I need to stop going to the worst-case scenario. I need to keep calm and ask questions to get the answers to deal with it rather than creating stories so that my mind spirals out of control.

12. What does this entire process tell you about the skills that need to be practiced or improved upon?

It tells me I need to basically practice every skill and that when everything happens all at once, makes it so bad.

CLIENT WORKSHEET

1. Identify (describe) an emotional trigger or a challenging situation.

2. What was the interaction with the other person?

3. How did you behave in the situation?

4. What were your thoughts about the trigger or situation?

5. What did you sense in your body (physical sensations)?

6. What emotions did you experience?

7. What did you imagine?

8. Indicate the firing order of the processes and what you notice first to the last (use the diagram).

9. Put the processes in order from which they bother you the most to the least?

10. What does this process tell you about yourself?

11. What do you need?

12. What does this entire process tell you about the skills that need to be practiced or improved upon?

Have your client continue to practice these skills. As they practice, they will get to know themselves better and feel more comfortable in their body. While it is important for your clients to get to know uncomfortable feelings and sensations and learn to cope through it, it is just as important to remind your clients that they also have powerful experiences.

Powerful Protectors for Emotional Resilience

Often individuals focus on their difficulties and may forget that they have strengths. They forget that they have worked through incredibly challenging situations in the past. This includes times they felt strong, confident, and empowered. Helping your client remember these experiences will help them recall major resources that can help them through more difficult times. It's a reminder for them that they have parts in them that are resilient and can be called upon when they need.

> Rachel: "I guess I don't ever talk about this, but I know I've been through a lot. I do have strength. I have been able to get through some really tough things. When I'm around others, like at work, they do look to me to handle the situations because I can compartmentalize the way I feel at work. I can do what needs to be done. Then I fall apart at home by myself, but I am able to get it together and others do depend on me."

Let's help your clients tap into their positive resources in the next exercise. They will create a symbol as a reminder for those positive qualities. They can use a tangible representation to carry with them as a reminder or they can keep it in their mind for referencing when needed in difficult times.

CLIENT EXERCISE: POWERFUL PROTECTORS

Can you think of a time either as a child or as an adult when things got really hard? How did you get through it? These times are easy to forget or downplay, reasoning it away like it wasn't a big deal—but it is! It doesn't matter how old you were when it happened or what the situation was—what matters most is that you realize that you have parts in you that are resilient, strong, confident, and powerful. In this next exercise, let's practice recalling those times.

Objective: Acknowledging resilience, strength, and confidence in yourself.
Directions: Complete the following exercise and use the symbol as a reminder of your positive qualities and strength.

Visualize a time when you felt completely confident, positive, empowered, and strong.

Describe the situation.

List the strengths that helped you get through the experience.

Where do you feel the positive feelings in your body?

Describe what the physical sensations feel like.

Can you think of an item (animal, object, idea, or quote) that best symbolizes your inherent qualities that got you through the situation? (For example, a tree, because you stood up for yourself and faced the challenge with confidence, or a lion, because you were able to show courage through a difficult time.)

How can you use this symbol as a reminder of your strengths during challenging times?

Now that your clients have some strategies for dealing with distress and difficult emotions, they may be more willing to practice these skills in relationships with others or participate in more social settings. Human connection is a fundamental need and a requirement for lasting eating disorder recovery. However, because of their past experiences, navigating social situations and relationships can be extremely challenging for our clients. Their psychosocial functioning has been compromised through avoidance and a multitude of other factors.

Rachel: "Okay, but even if I have the courage to hang out with my co-workers, I always feel there's more problems because I literally am not sure what to do in certain circumstances. It is so uncomfortable for me to tell others what I need. How do you even start doing that?"

The next chapter focuses on psychosocial functioning and the practical tools needed for eating disorder recovery in foundational skill #8 Using My Authentic Voice.

Bibliography

Algoe, S. B., Kurtz, L. E., & Grewen, K. (2017). Oxytocin and Social Bonds: The Role of Oxytocin in Perceptions of Romantic Partners' Bonding Behavior. *Psychological Science*. https://doi.org/10.1177/0956797617716922.

Arlt, J. et al. (2016). Contributions of cognitive inflexibility to eating disorder and social anxiety symptoms. *Eating Behaviors*, *21*, 30–32. https://doi.org/10.1016/j.eatbeh.2015.12.008.

Bardone-Cone, A. M., Lin, S. L., & Butler, R. M. (2017). Perfectionism and contingent self-worth in relation to disordered eating and anxiety. *Behavior Therapy*, *48*, 380–390. https://doi.org/10.1016/j.beth.2016.05.006.

Buchheim, A. et al.(2009). Oxytocin enhances the experience of attachment security. *Psychoneuroendocrinology*, *34*(9), 1417–1422. https://doi.org/10.1016/j.psyneuen.2009.04.002.

Dingemans, A., Danner, U., & Parks, M. (2017). Emotion Regulation in Binge Eating Disorder: A Review. *Nutrients*, *9*(11), 1274. DOI: 10.3390/nu9111274.

Foye, U., Hazlett, D. E., & Irving, P. (2019). "The body is a battleground for unwanted and unexpressed emotions": exploring eating disorders and the role of emotional intelligence. *Eating Disorders*, *27*(3), 321–342. https://doi.org/10.1080/10640266.2018.1517520.

Henderson, Z. B., Fox, J. R. E., Trayner, P., & Wittkowski, A. (2019). Emotional development in eating disorders: A qualitative metasynthesis. *Clinical Psychology & Psychotherapy*, *26*(4), 440–457. https://doi.org/10.1002/cpp.2365.

Leppanen, J. et al. (2022). The Role of Emotion Regulation in Eating Disorders: A Network Meta-Analysis Approach. *Frontiers in Psychiatry*, *13*, 793094. https://doi.org/10.3389/fpsyt.2022.793094.

Meneguzzo, P., Garolla, A., Bonello, E., & Todisco, P. (2022). Alexithymia, dissociation and emotional regulation in eating disorders: Evidence of improvement through specialized inpatient treatment. *Clinical Psychology & Psychotherapy*, *29*(2), 718–724. https://doi.org/10.1002/cpp.2665.

Momeñe, J. et al. (2022). Eating Disorders and Intimate Partner Violence: The Influence of Fear of Loneliness and Social Withdrawal. *Nutrients*, *14*(13), 2611. https://doi.org/10.3390/nu14132611.

Monell, E., Clinton, D., & Birgegård, A. (2018). Emotion dysregulation and eating disorders-Associations with diagnostic presentation and key symptoms. *The International Journal of Eating Disorders*, *51*(8), 921–930. https://doi.org/10.1002/eat.22925.

Monell, E., Clinton, D., & Birgegård, A. (2020). Self-directed behaviors differentially explain associations between emotion dysregulation and eating disorder psychopathology in patients with or without objective binge-eating. *Journal of Eating Disorders*, *8*, 17. https://doi.org/10.1186/s40337-020-00294-4.

Ortiz, A. M. L., Davis, H. A., Riley, E. N., & Smith, G. T. (2022). The interaction between affective lability and eating expectancies predicts binge eating. *Eating Disorders*, *30*(3), 331–344. https://doi.org/10.1080/10640266.2021.1905449.

Peláez-Fernández, M. A., Romero-Mesa, J., & Extremera, N. (2021). From Deficits in Emotional Intelligence to Eating Disorder Symptoms: A Sequential Path Analysis Approach Through Self-Esteem and Anxiety. *Frontiers in Psychology*,[Q10] 13:873073. doi: 10.3389/fpsyg.2022.873073.

Prefit, A. B., Cândea, D. M., & Szentagotai-Tătar, A. (2019). Emotion regulation across eating pathology: A meta-analysis. *Appetite*, *143*, 104438. DOI: 10.1016/j.appet.2019.104438.

Siegel, D. J. (2012). *The developing mind: How relationships and the brain interact to shape who we are* (2nd ed.). The Guilford Press

Vitale, E. M., & Smith, A. S. (2022). Neurobiology of Loneliness, Isolation, and Loss: Integrating Human and Animal Perspectives. *Frontiers in Behavioral Neuroscience*, *16*, 846315. https://doi.org/10.3389/fnbeh.2022.846315.

Chapter 10

Foundational Skill #8
Using My Authentic Voice

Individuals who struggle with eating disorders have challenges with *psychosocial functioning*. Psychosocial functioning is defined as the individual's ability to successfully interact with their environment, which includes establishing and sustaining satisfying relationships with family, significant others, friends and peers, appropriately handling responsibilities in their roles at school, work, and other social environments (Mehl et al. 2019). Studies show that psychological, emotional, and social challenges are the most predominant complications in people who struggle with eating disorders (Blodgett Salafia et al. 2015).

> *Rachel:* "*My anxiety gets really bad when I'm out in social situations. I feel like people are staring at me. I'm also scared that I'll upset someone. These days it seems people are short, and easily angered. I'm afraid someone will get angry at me. Then what do I do? It makes me anxious just thinking about it. It's hard for me at work too, but I force myself to do it.*"

As you can see in the example, Rachel has difficulty in her daily functioning around others. She struggles with social anxiety and fears being the object of others' anger. She has avoided social situations for years, fearing rejection and judgment from others, resulting in deficits in her social skills.

People who struggle with disordered eating struggle with social anxiety to such an extent that they are terrified of being seen—yet desperately want to be seen. Therefore, they agonize over expressing authenticity and showing others who they are. It is characteristic of individuals that struggle with disordered eating to possess traits of fear of rejection, needing to please others, conflict avoidant, shyness, and timidity; they also tend to have challenges with interpersonal sensitivity (Micali et al. 2017).

Because of these traits, they often encounter interpersonal problems (Arcelus et al. 2013) and are easily overwhelmed by their feelings. Their disordered eating behaviors become a coping mechanism to deal with the distress. People who struggle with eating disorders reported more frequent negative experiences and lower levels of psychological resilience that include less cohesion, harmony, tolerance, and more conflict in family relationships, leading to lower life satisfaction (Momeñe et al. 2022). These findings correlate with negative experiences and higher levels of loneliness (Matkovic et al. 2023).

Individuals commonly struggle with psychosocial impairments that include:

- **Public Self-consciousness and Social Anxiety:** They struggle with cognitive inflexibility which can affect levels of social anxiety and self-consciousness in public. Cognitive inflexibility represents their lack of awareness of options when unexpected situations arise. Their unwillingness or ability to adapt to changes makes it more challenging for them in social contexts. The inflexibility can partly be attributed to the fear of being seen negatively by others (Arlt et al. 2016).
- **Low Assertiveness**: Individuals struggle with feelings of helplessness, have a tendency to take on others' problems, a tendency to say "yes" to inappropriate demands and unreasonable requests—when they really want to say "no." They allow others to make decisions and speak for them even when they do not agree. They are challenged with speaking up for themselves and asserting boundaries with others (Forbush & Watson 2006).

DOI: 10.4324/9781032651408-15

- **Social Skill Deficits**: They have difficulty initiating and responding to the interactions of others, maintaining eye contact, being in the moment, are likely to misinterpret non-verbal cues, and struggle with situations that involve food or eating with others (MacIntyre et al. 2022).

In this chapter, we take a look at the importance of preventative interventions. These interventions involve social skills that teach your client presence, using their authentic voice, expressing their feelings and beliefs—and creating boundaries. These skills help with psychosocial functioning that helps to mitigate (Cardi et al. 2018):

- Loneliness.
- Poor interaction with peers and in social situations.
- Shyness: Defined as self-consciousness, negative self-preoccupation, low self-esteem, and fear of judgment and rejection.
- Anxiety and depression (feelings of hopelessness and helplessness).

When these issues are addressed they will have the ability to develop meaningful human connections for lasting eating disorder recovery.

Your clients will learn how their existing ways of interacting affects their relationships and social situations by:

- Understanding the origin of their communication style.
- Understanding the function of disordered eating and how it relates to communication.
- Understanding communication styles.
- Understanding how their beliefs affect their communication.
- Effectively creating and applying boundaries in their relationships.

Communication in the Family of Origin

Communication is first learned in the family of origin. It is modeled by members of the family from the moment one is born. For example, we watched our mother and father discuss issues, work through misunderstandings, engage in disagreements and ultimately how they communicate when resolving conflict. These observations contribute to the understanding about how to communicate with others. Further, daily interactions with family members can reinforce our clients' decision to choose faulty but protective ways of communicating. For example:

> Rachel: "I never had a problem asking for what I need when I was younger. I remember asking for my mom to stay with me because I was scared. I remember asking to spend time with my dad. Their response was usually something like, 'Ok, sure.' But then, they ignore me, and they don't follow through and then when I asked again, they would say, 'What is wrong with you? You are so needy. I stopped asking.'"

This is a common example in families with individuals that struggle with eating. Often as children they recognized what they needed and may have directly asked for it—but their requests may have been ignored, punished, or rejected—therefore, they learned to refrain from voicing their needs as a way to protect themselves. In the next exercise, your clients will explore the origin of their communication style. This will help them understand the function of their disordered eating.

Families may have their own unique, or cultural beliefs and values that they reinforce about communication. For example, in some cultures children are taught to be passive, and never argue with others. Therefore, individuals may perceive any disagreement as conflict or an argument waiting to happen. It could stir up past negative experiences of explosive anger and therefore they tend to avoid any conflict all together. This reinforces passive communication—and prevents them from getting their needs met—continuing unhelpful eating behaviors to cope with their unsettled feelings.

CLIENT WORKSHEET: AWARENESS OF COMMUNICATION

Have you ever wondered why it is difficult for you to speak up? Have you wondered what could happen if you were able to communicate more effectively? Let's explore how your family's interactions influence your communication style in your relationships.

Objective: Gain awareness about learned patterns of communication.
Directions: Complete the following worksheet and discuss with your therapist.

How did your family members communicate with one another?

How did you communicate your needs to your family members? How did they respond?

How did your family members ask for what they needed? What did you notice about the way they communicated?

How do you tend to communicate your needs with your family and with others?

How do you communicate your beliefs or values when you disagree with someone in your family? How about with others?

Disordered eating can have many functions as you have seen in previous chapters which means treating and helping your client completely recover from an eating disorder can be complex and challenging. Maladaptive eating can function as a form of communication. Let's take a look at what that means.

The Language of Disordered Eating

When individuals are unable to articulate their feelings, needs, or wants they suppress it. They learned that it is undesirable for them to express their needs, therefore it doesn't feel safe nor acceptable for them to directly ask for what they desire. They may have been rejected in their attempts in the past and have learned to use maladaptive coping in order to deal with their distress. Eventually, their eating behaviors become a way for them to communicate feelings, needs, and wants—without having to use verbal expression, thereby avoiding blatant rejection.

For example:

Rachel: "I do remember thinking when I was younger, if I just skipped dinner, then my mom would know I was mad at her. She would realize that something is wrong."

In the past, when Rachel had verbally expressed her needs her parents hadn't acknowledged her so she resorted to abstaining from dinner. Unfortunately, these subtle behaviors usually go unnoticed too. Often this can be the start of problematic eating behaviors. Over time, weight loss is noticeable—and may then be reinforced inadvertently.

Rachel: "I recall losing a few pounds after not eating for several days. My mom never noticed. But everyone else did at school. I remember I was 13 when I started dating Jeremy. It felt good. But I remember thinking, 'He likes me because I am skinny.'"

In this example, though she failed to get her mom's attention, Rachel associated her weight loss with a positive event—being noticed, accepted, and loved. The culture of the "thin ideal" reinforces her experience and her beliefs.

Your client may have limited awareness about what they are communicating through their behaviors with food. However, when they are introduced and encouraged to view their eating disorder behaviors from a different perspective—such as how the behavior functions in their lives. They are then able to identify what initiated the eating disorder behavior and recall elements that they had forgotten. They are able to make connections more easily and recognize that these functions are actually pretty common—and that they are not alone in engaging in these behaviors for these reasons. For example:

> Rachel: "I had no idea there were so many reasons why I use eating behaviors. I never thought about my eating behaviors this way, but having questions posed to me in this way helps me realize that this is a thing, that others have a hard time saying how they feel too, and it feels like we can only say it through what we do with food."

Use the exercises in Chapter 4 in conjunction with the exercises in this chapter to help your cleitns to decode the metaphor behind their behaviors with food.

Let's take a look at how your client has been communicating through their eating disorder behaviors.

RACHEL'S WORKSHEET: INCREASING AWARENESS OF FOOD BEHAVIORS

Describe a food behavior (ritual) that you do while eating?	What happens if you stop using that behavior (ritual)?	What do you think the behavior (ritual) represents?	How do you feel this behavior (ritual) helps you with your current situation? Or represents a current situation?
I drink a glass of water before I even start to eat.	I tried but I feel empty. I feel like I'll have to eat more.	It represents my fear that I will eat too much, if I don't first get full off of water.	It helps me with my anxiety and fear. I know I have a lot of anxiety with everything I'm going through.
I put hot sauce all over my food if it's something that I really like.	I feel scared and out of control because I feel like I have no will power to stop eating.	I feel like I have to sabotage something like putting hot sauce on food. I don't even like hot sauce, out of fear I won't have the ability to stop.	It represents all my relationships. Whenever I like someone, I feel like I need to sabotage it because I feel like I can't control my feelings and I'll get hurt.

CLIENT WORKSHEET: INCREASING AWARENESS OF FOOD BEHAVIORS

Have you ever noticed that you may engage in certain behaviors when you eat? For example, you may cut food into small pieces, over indulge in condiments, or push food around on your plate. Did you know that there is meaning behind these behaviors? The behaviors can communicate what you may be feeling, your desires, wants, or needs that you have not been able to express. When you are aware that these behaviors are a way of communicating then you can explore your needs and better understand why you are compelled to engage in eating in this way.

Objective: Uncover and gain awareness about food behaviors and what they are communicating.
Directions: Complete this exercise when you are exploring more about the eating behaviors you are actively engaging in. Complete the questions and discuss your responses with your therapist.

Describe a food behavior or ritual that you do while eating	What happens if you stop using that behavior or ritual?	What do you think the behavior or ritual represents?	How do you feel this behavior or ritual helps you with your current situation? Or represents a current situation?

As you can see in Rachel's completed exercise, her food behaviors are communicating her feelings. When your client learns that they are communicating when they are engaging in eating disorder behaviors, they can then practice identifying what their true needs are, and will be able to address those feelings in psychotherapy. They are then able to practice their communication skills to ask for what they need instead of communicating through their eating behaviors.

Now let's help your clients understand what their eating behaviors are conveying and help them to identify how they can verbally communicate their needs instead.

RACHEL'S WORKSHEET: COMMUNICATION THROUGH EATING DISORDER BEHAVIORS

Describe a time you were aware that you were using an eating disorder behavior. What was the situation and the eating disorder behavior used?	What were you communicating?	How did you want others to respond?	What did you need, want, desire?	What could you have said instead?
I was with Mom, and it was the first time she asked me why I didn't eat. I restricted more that night. I don't think I ate anything.	*I was communicating anger. I felt really powerful that she finally cared.*	*I wanted her to respond by caring what happens to me. By asking me how I was doing. To show me she cared.*	*I didn't want her to stop giving me attention. And I wanted to push her away and I wanted her to still care. I wanted her to convince me that she cares about me and loves me.*	*I guess I could have told her how I felt. But I feel like I have so many times and she didn't hear me. I feel it's more powerful when I just show her.*

Describe a time you were aware that you were using an eating disorder behavior. What was the situation and the eating disorder behavior used?	What were you communicating?	How did you want others to respond?	What did you need, want, desire?	What could you have said instead?
I was with my boyfriend, and I asked him to pick up something I needed from the store. He told me he forgot and didn't pick it up. I was so angry. I didn't eat that night.	*Anger. I was so angry. I was communicating to him that I was angry at him. And because he couldn't do what I asked, it affected my ability to eat. I wanted to show him how he affects me. I wanted to punish him.*	*I wanted him to apologize and show me that my needs matter.*	*I wanted him to care and realize my needs are important. I wanted him take care of me.*	*I guess I could have told him how hurt I was and told him how it made me feel.*

CLIENT EXERCISE: COMMUNICATION THROUGH ED BEHAVIORS

Have you ever eaten a whole bag of chips after a very stressful day at school or work? Or lost your appetite completely even though you were hungry a few minutes before? When we reach for food (or restrict it) to cope when feeling upset, sad, nervous, excited, or any other emotion, it isn't a cause for alarm once in a while, but it can be a problem when it's your primary way of coping. What feelings are your eating behaviors expressing? Let's find out.

Objective: Create awareness about what eating disorder behaviors are communicating.
Directions: Complete the worksheet below and discuss with your therapist. See Rachel's completed example.

Describe eating disorder behavior.	What are you communicating?	How do you want others to respond?	What do you need, want, desire?	What can you say instead?

Describe eating disorder behavior.	What are you communicating?	How do you want others to respond?	What do you need, want, desire?	What can you say instead?

Communication Styles

People communicate in various ways and this can affect the individual's urges to utilize maladaptive coping tools because it often brings up uncomfortable and unsettling emotions, specifically when communication is ineffective and negatively impacts their relationships. For example:

Rachel: "I'm usually passive and avoid conflict. But when I can't handle it anymore, when I'm angry, I explode and say mean things to someone I care about. I'm frustrated. Of course, they're upset with me. Then I have guilt and anxiety for what I did. I usually binge and tell myself that I'm such a horrible loser."

Rachel's style of communication is usually passive and avoidant—however, when she isn't able to suppress her emotions, she can become explosive and aggressive (Ioannou & Fox 2009.). This is consistent with both how she handles her feelings and how she learned to communicate at an early age.

Let's briefly review communication styles:

- Passive: People with passive communication styles avoid directly expressing what they feel or think. They often let others decide and find it difficult to stand up for themselves.
- Passive-Aggressive: Passive-aggressive communication is expressing dislike and or negative thoughts indirectly rather than openly. For example, when someone is angry, they behave and speak as if everything were fine, but they may express negativity about the person to a third party.
- Aggressive: Aggressive communication is expressed by yelling, shouting, blaming, using hostility, demanding, or being verbally abusive.
- Assertive: Assertive communication is honoring the individual's own thoughts and feelings while honoring the other person at the same time—by not putting themselves or the other person down.

Let's take a look at your how your clients tend to communicate.

CLIENT EXERCISE: COMMUNICATION QUIZ

When it comes to communicating, we all have different styles, and we may respond differently in various situations. Let's take a quick quiz to get an idea of your primary communication style and whether you might need help to communicate more effectively.

Objective: Create awareness of your communication style and identify tendencies that need to be addressed. Directions:

1. Complete the quiz by circling or writing down your answers to each question.
2. When you're finished, add up the total number of As, Bs, Cs, and Ds. Check your responses with the key at the end of the quiz.
3. Answer the Reflection Questions at the end, and share the results with your therapist if you like.

---

1. If someone cuts in front of you in line, which of the following best reflects what you'd likely say:

   A) Nothing, because I don't want to make a scene.
   B) Think to yourself, "They are so rude." But smile at them and later tell everyone about it.
   C) "Hey! There's a line cutter here!"
   D) "Excuse me, I'm also in line."

2. You need to prepare for a party and need help with cooking. Which of the following are you most likely to say as you head into the kitchen?
   A) "There's so much I need to do. I hope I can cook everything myself before everyone gets here."
   B) Feel really angry but say, "I'm fine. You all just relax. I will take care of it."
   C) "I'm doing this alone! Let's just cancel the party since no one wants to help!"
   D) "Could you please help. I can't possibly do all of this myself."

3. You're at a restaurant and they mixed up your order. The food is okay but not something you would normally order. How would you most likely handle it?
   A) Just eat it anyway because you don't want to draw attention to yourself.
   B) Feel upset, but say, "No problem." And then be angry for the rest of the day.
   C) Demand for them to get your order right and give it to you for free since they messed up.
   D) Tell the waiter that your order is incorrect and reorder.

4. You're out with your friends and they make plans for the night you disagree with. What are you most likely to do?
   A) Say nothing because everyone else likes the idea.
   B) Think to yourself "I'm never doing this again." But smile and pretend you're having fun.
   C) Tell them they're insane and leave.
   D) Express how you feel about the plans as clearly as possible.

5. You're at work but on a 30-minute lunch break. Your mother calls, asking you to come over right away to help her with her computer. What are you most likely to do?
   A) Head to your mom's and skip lunch.
   B) Tell her, "I'm on my way" knowing you're not. Then just ignore her calls.
   C) Tell your mom you're not an on-call technician and has to figure it out on her own.
   D) Tell your mom you are at work and can come by when you're done.

6. You overhear another student saying that she doesn't like you in her group because you're difficult to work with. What are you be most likely to do?
   A) Say nothing, because you just want to disappear.
   B) Think to yourself, "Just you wait and see how difficult I can make your life."

C) Stare at the student, "Do you want to make things more difficult?"
D) Wait until you can speak to the student alone and ask if you can talk about it.

7. You are having trouble with your landscaper. Your partner asks your opinion about how to resolve it. What are you most likely to say?
   A) "I have no idea. What do you want to do?"
   B) "It was your idea to hire the landscaper. I don't have a problem!"
   C) "Every landscaper is horrible. This is your problem, deal with it."
   D) "Can we talk to the landscaper to find a compromise?"

8. You order a combination pizza and they forgot the vegetables on the pizza. What are you most likely to do?
   A) Take the pizza home and hope your family doesn't notice.
   B) Tell the clerk everything is fine and then write a complaint about the clerk.
   C) "What the heck, this is not a combo! I demand a combo."
   D) Let them know that you ordered a combo to get the order corrected.

9. Your co-worker's been out sick and you've been covering for him. Now he is going on vacation. What are you most likely to do?
   A) Just cover for him again even if you don't want to.
   B) Tell your co-worker, "You are really selfish."
   C) "So, you're going on vacation again? Good luck, I'm not covering you."
   D) Tell him, "Sounds like you're really excited. Unfortunately, I won't be able to cover again and maybe you may need to find another back up."

10. On your birthday, your friend forgets to wish you a happy birthday—your feelings are hurt. What are you most likely to say?
    A) Nothing, it shouldn't matter anyway.
    B) "I knew she would forget." And then avoid her.
    C) "Boy, this is terrible. I can't believe I even call her a friend!"
    D) "She must've been really busy, and I can just call her and ask if she wants to hang out."

11. You forgot to feed your dog. Your spouse confronts you angrily about it. What are you most likely to do/say?
    A) Just ignore him. But tell him you didn't hear him.
    B) Tell your friends, "My spouse is a jerk."
    C) "From now on you feed your damn dog."
    D) "You're right. I forgot to feed our dog. In the future, if you notice it, could you just feed him?"

Total As_____Total Bs_____Total Cs_____Total Ds_____
Take your highest score above to find your communication style.

Note: If you have two scores that are high and very close in number, this means you probably use both styles as needed.

Mostly As: Your primary communication style is passive.
Mostly Bs: Your primary communication style is passive-aggressive.
Mostly Cs: Your primary communication style is aggressive.
Mostly Ds: Your primary communication style is assertive.

Reflection Questions

12. How do you feel/think about your results? Do you feel/think your results are accurate? Why or why not?

13. How do you feel/think your communication style has affected your relationships, and social situations?

14. Which communication style do you feel would be most effective for you?

15. How would you like to improve on your communication style?

How Beliefs Impact Communication Styles

Individuals may have a tendency to communicate in ineffective ways due to the negative core beliefs they hold. For example, your client may have the core belief that they should please others, therefore, they may go along with something they disagree with because they desperately want to be liked by others. They will be passive in articulating their needs so it may appear as though they are okay with the situation, but they are not. If these patterns are not addressed and identified as problematic, your clients will continue to communicate in these ineffective ways reinforcing challenges in their psychosocial functioning, resulting in isolation, and social anxiety. Let's take a look at some examples of how these communication styles can cause challenges in relationships.

Passive and Passive Aggressive Communication

Rachel: "I have to do things for others in order to feel valued or worthy."
"If people care about me, they should already know what I need. I shouldn't have to ask."

Example #1: "I was invited to a friend's house for dinner. I found myself cleaning up and no one helped. I felt so used—and I didn't ask anyone for any help. I was in the kitchen for the entire party. I thought I should be helpful. I couldn't help feeling sad and disappointed that no one came to check on me. If they really cared about me, don't you think, they would have come to check in on me? This is why I don't like hanging out with people. I feel horrible afterwards and just ate until my stomach hurt when I got home."

In this example, Rachel believes that in order to be worthy she has to be useful. Therefore, she was unable to enjoy the dinner party as a guest. Her beliefs were further reinforced because she was unable to ask for help. She felt sad, used, and disappointed because she felt alone. Her friends didn't know that she felt that way. However, this is a common pattern for Rachel. She feels the need to be helpful but it results in resentful feelings towards others.

Rachel: "I would rather let others make the decision. Then when something goes wrong, I'm not to be blamed for the decision. And I can be upset that they made the wrong decision."

Example #2: "We worked in groups a lot at school. I disagreed with my group, but never told them. I just went along with what they all wanted. When we received our grades, it wasn't so good. I felt upset with them because they made wrong decisions. I don't speak up because at least I know I'm not to be blamed and I would rather they be wrong. This is another reason I don't like being around others. We will disagree. I just can't deal with being blamed or at fault for making the wrong decision."

In example #2, Rachel's passive communication is a way to protect herself from feeling like a failure. It is also protection from potentially being blamed for any mistakes. She would rather others make decisions so that she doesn't have to take responsibility or deal with any negative consequences such as the group's judgments about her. This reinforces her fear to speak up and reinforces her doubt that people will accept her for beliefs and for who she is.

Aggressive Communication

Rachel: "I have to be aggressive for others to hear me."

Example #1: *"I asked my boyfriend to please take out the garbage, and he sits and ignores me. He's playing with his video game and just tuning me out. I get so angry. I yell on the top of my lungs for him to pay attention to me and then I turn off his game. Oh, he gets really upset with me. In that moment, I'm so angry. I can't stop."*

In this example, Rachel feels ignored by her boyfriend. She believes that she has to become aggressive in order for him to actually listen to her. She has difficulty communicating what she needs, and her boyfriend has learned to tune her out. This reinforces the pattern of negative communication.

Rachel: "They'll all think I'm weak."

Example #2: *"When I am sad, I was made fun of. My mom and dad would make comments and call me silly. If I asked for what I needed in a calm voice, they would ignore me. If I cried watching a movie, they would make fun of me and tell I me I was weak. When I am angry, they tend to listen. But I am so tired of being angry, so I don't say anything at all. I get frustrated and have been acting out by throwing things."*

Rachel struggles with showing her feelings and asking for what she needs because she was judged and ridiculed as being weak by her family. Therefore, Rachel adopted their belief that showing feelings of sadness and hurt are considered weak. Her family reinforced Rachel's aggressive acting out behaviors because they were more likely to pay attention to her when she behaved in that way. This is the reason Rachel has a tendency to swing between a passive communication style to an aggressive communication style.

In the next exercise, your clients will explore their communication style and how their negative core beliefs in impact the one way they communicate.

Therapist Tip:

- *Be sure to go over negative core beliefs with your client before the next exercise.*

CLIENT WORKSHEET: EXPLORING YOUR COMMUNICATION STYLE

Your negative core beliefs impact your communication style. When your beliefs are tied into the way you communicate, it can be more challenging. However, when you can identify how your beliefs around communication have been affecting your relationships, you will be able to separate your negative beliefs from your current situation and practice communication more effectively.

Objective: Increase awareness around current communication style and how affects you.
Directions: Complete worksheet and discuss with your therapist.

What are your beliefs about a passive (passive-aggressive) communication style?

How does using a passive, passive-aggressive communication style affect your relationships?

How does using a passive, passive-aggressive communication style affect your maladaptive eating behaviors?

Individuals who struggle with eating often need to learn assertiveness skills. They have difficulty with direct communication because they misinterpret it as aggression. They fear that others will be upset, reject, or judge them. They experience shame for expressing themselves having learned at a young age that disagreeing with others can have a negative result. They often feel stuck because expressing their feelings, needs, and wants have been shut down for so long. They feel guilty for speaking up for themselves—and are not sure how to begin practicing assertiveness.

The next exercise helps your clients to practice assertiveness communication by giving them structure and a formula to practice. As your clients become more comfortable with communicating assertively, this will become more natural for them.

CLIENT WORKSHEET: ASSERTIVENESS COMMUNICATION

You may recognize that you need to practice clarity and directness in the way you communicate. This can be challenging for you, and you may not know where to begin. This exercise can help you to practice expressing your feelings and asking for what you need.

Objective: Practice assertiveness using the assertiveness formula.
Directions: Complete the following worksheet, and practice applying assertiveness formula to real life situations.

The assertiveness formula looks like this:

I feel __[emotion: sad, angry, upset]_____ **when you __** [behavior that you are addressing]
_____**and I wish (you/we) could**
__[your request]_____.

Example:

Rachel: "My co-worker hasn't checked with me to see whether or not I was available to cover her shift. They just scheduled me to cover for her and I don't want to do it. I don't have a good excuse. I just don't want to work tomorrow".

Assertiveness formula example:

*"I feel **frustrated**, when you **schedule me to work without first checking,** and I wish you **would check with me before assigning me to work on my day off."***

---

1. Describe a situation that's challenging for you that involves another person.

2. How do you feel about the situation?

3. What behavior or action is occurring that you would like to address?

4. What would make the situation better? What request would you like to make?

5. Using the information from questions 1–4, write an assertiveness statement using the formula.

The assertiveness formula will also be effective for individuals learning to establish boundaries with others. When your client can identify their ineffective communication style and understand what kept them from speaking directly to others, they will also likely report not having learned how to establish appropriate boundaries which causes anxiety in unpredictable social situations. This is one reason that individuals have difficulty in social scenarios and problems in interpersonal relationships.

Boundary Setting

Creating boundaries can be challenging especially for those who did not have appropriate boundaries in their family of origin. When poor boundaries have been normalized—and intrusive behaviors have been viewed as acceptable—our clients will tend to use their eating disorder behaviors to create the boundaries that they need. This becomes another functional aspect of disordered eating. Some individuals clearly recognize they are using the eating disorder behaviors for this reason, while others have limited awareness and need to explore and address underlying issues.

For example: Individuals that struggle with maladaptive eating behaviors have shared the following statements about how their eating disorder behaviors as an attempt to construct boundaries with others. The example statements below show the kind of boundary the individual needed, how the eating disorder functions as a boundary, and what they needed to communicate instead of use their eating disorder. This is important because often our clients are not aware that they are doing this, however, when this brought to their attention, they can recognize how their eating disorder has been functional in an effort to establish a boundary.

How an Eating Disorder Functions in Establishing Boundaries

Example #1 *Physical Space Boundary*

Eating disorder function:

- *"I feel protected and safe when I'm in a bigger body. People can get too close to me, and I noticed that when I'm bigger, it helps keep them at a distance."*

Assertive communication of needed boundary:

- *"I just need some physical space, so I'll take a few steps back."*

Example #2 *Emotional Boundary*

Eating disorder function:

- *"When I'm not eating, people see me as fragile, delicate. I feel that people treat me kinder. They are not as hard on me and there's less pressure for me to do what they ask. They don't expect me to take care of them as much. They view me as sick. I would rather they view me as sick then as a failure that can't do what they need me to do."*

Assertive communication of needed boundary:

- *"There's a lot I am dealing with right now and cannot be of support to you. I will let you know what I can do if things change and things become more manageable."*

Example #3 *Intellectual Boundary:*

Eating disorder function:

- *"I have a lot of boundaries around my food—like what I can have, and when I can have it. I also have boundaries around the positioning of food on my plate. I need to control everything, what I eat, my weight, what I do, basically all of it. I hate it. At least people can't tell me what to eat and how to eat. People are always telling me what to think or how to think."*

Assertive communication of needed boundary:

- *"Thank you for your opinion. I prefer not to discuss this any further. If I need something I will let you know."*

In these examples, manipulating their food and eating becomes their way of communicating what they need from others. This prevents clear communication and healthy relationships. An antidote is assertive communication. By practicing the assertiveness formula in their communication, individuals can create healthy boundaries. When they are using their authentic voice there will be no need to use food behaviors or their body to communicate their need for boundaries.

There are various types of boundaries that individuals who struggle with disordered eating commonly have difficulty with. When your client can identify their challenges, it can help them gain more clarity on how they can use the assertiveness formula to practice effective boundary setting.

Let's briefly review a few of the boundaries that your client may have challenges with, along with sample questions that your clients can ask themselves so that they gain awareness and will be able to recognize when they may need to practice asserting boundaries.

CLIENT WORKSHEET: TYPES OF BOUNDARIES

When someone violates any of your personal boundaries it may be difficult to recognize at first. You may notice an icky sensation in your body, or you may notice anger surfacing. Sometimes the problem is not even realizing that your boundaries were encroached on. Did you know that there are different types of boundaries? Recognizing that there are various types of boundaries can help you clarify how you may need to practice asserting boundaries.

Objective: Gain awareness of types of boundaries and practice creating boundaries.
Directions: Complete the questions below and discuss with your therapist.

- **Physical Boundaries**: This is a boundary that protects your body and your physical space. It allows you the right to privacy and the right not to be touched.

  Questions to ask yourself:

  - How comfortable am I with physical closeness, such as handshakes, hugs, and/or touch?
  - How comfortable am I with sharing my physical space (in public and in private spaces)?

  Describe a situation where you felt your boundary was overstepped.

  What can you say or do to establish a physical boundary?

- **Emotional Boundaries**: This is a boundary that allows you the right to your own feelings—and being accountable for your own feelings. This boundary helps to differentiate your feelings from the feelings of others and to not take on the responsibility to care for others' feelings. It helps you to practice emotional safety by not oversharing personal information with people where trust hasn't been established.

  Questions to ask yourself:

  - What are you comfortable sharing with others about yourself? With whom?
  - How do I not emotionally "dump" on others? How do I respond when others come to me with an emotional "dump"?

  Describe a situation where you felt your emotional boundary was overstepped.

  What can you say or do to establish an emotional boundary?

- **Time Boundaries**: This boundary means honoring and having respect for your own time as well as someone else's. Some people consistently show up late for appointments, or you may have difficulty with people who are constantly taking up your time or volunteering your time to others.

  Questions to ask yourself:

  - How much time do I need for myself today?
  - How long am I willing to wait for someone who is consistently late?

  Describe a situation where you felt your time boundary was overstepped.

  What can you say or do to establish a time boundary?

- **Sexual Boundaries:** Sexual boundaries include your physical and emotional boundaries. This boundary also includes acceptable language, information, and/or ideas about sexuality. This means having a clear understanding and enforcing the sexual boundaries for you and your partner around consent. This means only "yes" means yes!

  Questions to ask yourself:

  - What types of sexual intimacy am I comfortable with?
  - How do I communicate consent with my partner?

  Describe a situation where you felt your sexual boundaries were overstepped.

  What can you say or do to establish a sexual boundary?

- **Intellectual Boundaries:** This is a boundary is pertaining to your thoughts and your beliefs. You have a right to your own thoughts, ideas, opinions, and wishes.

  Questions to ask yourself:

  - How will I show others I respect their ideas and perspectives?
  - What does respecting ideas and perspectives mean to me?

  Describe a situation where you felt your intellectual boundaries were overstepped.

  What can you say or do to establish an intellectual boundary?

- **Material/Financial Boundaries:** This boundary protects your financial resources and possessions. You have the right to decide how you would like to spend your resources or how you would like to share your possessions. You are not obligated to financially take care of someone else who is not your dependent.

  Questions to ask yourself.

  - What can I afford to share?
  - How would this affect me if I share or I lend out my resources and it is not returned?

  Describe a situation where you felt your material/ financial boundaries were overstepped.

  What can you say or do to establish a material/financial boundary?

Now that your client is aware of the various types of boundaries, let's take a look at their experiences with boundaries and how it relates to their eating disorder behaviors.

CLIENT WORKSHEET: THE IMPACT OF BOUNDARIES

The ability to create personal boundaries is an essential skill for lasting eating disorder recovery. At first, it may be a little challenging but with practice it will become easier and feel more natural. Let's take a look at how boundary setting impacts you.

Objective: Learn the importance of boundaries and how they impact you.
Directions: Complete the worksheet below and discuss with your therapist.

---

1. What has your experience been with appropriate boundary setting?

2. What have you noticed in your relationships with family and friends, and relationships with your boundaries?

3. How do you feel your food behaviors are related to your ability to establish boundaries?

4. How do you feel your body image or weight is related to your ability to establish boundaries?

5. How do you feel your ability to establish boundaries with others will change your perspective about taking risks in social scenarios?

6. What has been your story about your ability to develop healthy relationships, function in social situations, and be able to share what you believe (your truth) with others?

In the next foundational skill, we take a look at how your client's story—their experiences, thoughts, feelings, identity, and how their eating disorder keeps them stuck. The last foundational skill #9 *Changing My Story* addresses your client's identity, purpose, motivations, desires, wants, needs, and passions. They hold on to an outdated version of themselves and have been repeating the same old unhelpful story and they will need to learn this to shed their eating disorder identity and let go of the parts that no longer benefit them. They can do this by accepting and healing their past—by moving on—and editing their life story.

Bibliography

Arcelus, J., Haslam, M., Farrow, C., & Meyer, C. (2013). The role of interpersonal functioning in the maintenance of eating psychopathology: a systematic review and testable model. *Clinical Psychology Review*, *33*(1), 156–167. https://doi.org/10.1016/j.cpr.2012.10.009.

Arlt, J. et al. (2016). Contributions of cognitive inflexibility to eating disorder and social anxiety symptoms. *Eating Behaviors*, *21*, 30–32. https://doi.org/10.1016/j.eatbeh.2015.12.008.

Blodgett Salafia, E. H. et al. (2015). Perceptions of the causes of eating disorders: a comparison of individuals with and without eating disorders. *Journal of Eating Disorders*, *3*, 32. https://doi.org/10.1186/s40337-015-0069-8.

Cardi, V., Tchanturia, K., & Treasure, J. (2018). Premorbid and Illness-related Social Difficulties in Eating Disorders: An Overview of the Literature and Treatment Developments. *Current neuropharmacology*, *16*(8), 1122–1130. https://doi.org/10.2174/1570159X16666180118100028.

Forbush, K., & Watson, D. (2006). Emotional inhibition and personality traits: A comparison of women with anorexia, bulimia, and normal controls. *Annals of Clinical Psychiatry*, *18*(2), 115–121. https://doi.org/10.1080/10401230600614637.

Ioannou, K., & Fox, J. R. (2009). Perception of threat from emotions and its role in poor emotional expression within eating pathology. *Clinical Psychology & Psychotherapy*, *16*(4), 336–347. https://doi.org/10.1002/cpp.632.

MacIntyre, R. I. et al. (2021). Measurement of the influences of social processes in appetite using ecological momentary assessment. *Appetite*, *161*, 105126. https://doi.org/10.1016/j.appet.2021.105126.

Matkovic, H., Brajkovic, L., & Kopilaš, V. (2023). Psychosocial Factors of Subjective Well-Being in Women with Eating Disorders. *Behavioral Sciences*, *13*(7), 594. http://dx.doi.org/10.3390/bs13070594.

Mehl, A., Rohde, P., Gau, J. M., & Stice, E. (2019). Disaggregating the predictive effects of impaired psychosocial functioning on future DSM-5 eating disorder onset in high-risk female adolescents. *The International Journal of Eating Disorders*, *52*(7), 817–824. https://doi.org/10.1002/eat.23082.

Micali, N. et al. (2017). Lifetime and 12-month prevalence of eating disorders amongst women in mid-life: a population-based study of diagnoses and risk factors. *BMC Medicine*, *15*(1), 12. https://doi.org/10.1186/s12916-016-0766-4.

Momeñe, J. et al. (2022). Eating Disorders and Intimate Partner Violence: The Influence of Fear of Loneliness and Social Withdrawal. *Nutrients*, *14*(13), 2611. https://doi.org/10.3390/nu14132611.

Part V

Teaching Existential Skills for Recovery

Chapter 11

Foundational Skill #9
Changing My Story

Individuals who struggle with eating have a narrative that they've been repeating to themselves for years. Unfortunately, this narrative consists of their negative experiences and beliefs. Since they look for their beliefs to be reinforced by their experiences it's often challenging for them to go outside of their comfort zone to create new experiences to replace their old narrative. They have replayed unhelpful thoughts and internalized old beliefs about who they are, what they deserve, and ultimately their story about their eating disorder recovery.

> *Rachel: "I can practice all these skills and sometimes I still find myself with urges to use behaviors. I get so discouraged and I tell myself, maybe eating disorder recovery isn't possible for me. Maybe I will always have an eating disorder and that's just part of who I am."*

The many functions of the eating disorder and the underlying issues that accompany eating behaviors make it difficult to relinquish. Therefore, it is important to identify any areas that are still affected by the disordered behaviors, areas that are keeping individuals stuck in the need to keep their eating disorder.

But what if their eating disorder has been a part of their life for so long that it has become a part of their identity?

Often individuals consider having an eating disorder as part of their identity (Ison & Kent 2010). Therefore, in order for your client to fully let go of their eating disorder, they need to understand how they may still be affected by an identity with having an eating disorder (McNamara & Parsons 2016). Are there any beneficial secondary gains in maintaining their eating disorder?

> *Rachel: "When I was in high school, I avoided school dances because I was afraid that no one would invite me to the dance. People assumed I didn't go because I was too sick to go. No one ever asked if I had a date. It helped me feel better that people just thought it was because I was sick, not because no one invited me."*

In this example, having an eating disorder gives Rachel a reason for not participating in social events. People just assumed that Rachel was too sick to attend and never questioned her. Therefore, Rachel feels protected and can avoid the feelings of discomfort from others asking if she was invited to the dance. This is her way of protecting herself from the possibility of social rejection and others knowing about it.

Individuals also have to explore their identity outside of their eating disorder. Who are they without their eating disorder? What else has their eating disorder protected them from? This is common since individuals who've have had their eating disorder for years may have forgotten about aspects that made up who they were before the eating disorder's stronghold took effect. Their eating disorder serves as part of their identity—a protective factor—as a justifiable reason for their avoidance of life. For example:

> *Rachel: "I didn't compete in the school debate team. It was for speech class. I got an excuse for not attending because everyone knew I was sick. Everyone knows I had an eating disorder and no one questioned it. I secretly didn't want to compete because I feared failing. I'd rather be known as Rachel, the girl with an eating disorder, then Rachel the failure, loser."*

DOI: 10.4324/9781032651408-17

In this example Rachel's eating disorder is functioning as a part of her identity. The eating disorder identity allows Rachel to avoid any situation that she fears. The function of the eating disorder protects her from any risk of perceived humiliation, judgment, and or embarrassment that she could be vulnerable to if she was living her life fully—taking on normal challenges that could result in mistakes and/or failures.

In this chapter, we focus on healing old outdated beliefs, identifying individual's values, that gives them meaning in their lives. This includes their passions, pursuits, motivations—the ability to recognize their strengths, and gifts so that they are able to change their story about who they are and to identify what they want for their future, free from their old eating disorder story. In order to do this, individuals will practice and cultivate this skill through exercises and completing worksheets to enable them to:

- Identify old beliefs and secondary gains from their eating disorder.
- Empower themselves to edit and make changes to their stories.
- Identify meaning, purpose, and significance in their lives.
- Look to future legacy and goals.
- Use tools and activities that support a new story.
- Apply behavioral changes and practice new activities.
- Understand the importance of connection in changing their recovery story.

Identifying Old Beliefs and Secondary Gains from Eating Disorders

Even though most people who struggle with disordered eating want to progress and live their lives free from their eating disorder, change in general can feel overwhelming and bring on uneasy feelings (Ferrier-Auerbach & Martens 2009). Therefore, it is important to address this apprehension and help individuals understand that change, even if positive, can be uncomfortable. Individuals have shared some example statements below that make them wary of letting go of their eating disorder altogether because they had been benefiting from it being part of their identities. These old eating disorder beliefs and secondary gains can keep individuals stuck in old patterns if it not addressed.

"My eating disorder has been my best friend for all of the past years and it has always been there for me. If I'm angry at someone at work, I immediately think about how nice it will be to get home, and eat my ice cream on the couch alone in peace. I get excited just thinking about it."

Secondary gain: As a comforting friend.

"My belief has always been—Who needs friends, when you have food that doesn't judge you?"

"What would I do with all the time that I have? I'd feel like something is missing. I'm constantly thinking about food, preparing it, looking at recipes, and watching shows on what I can make next. I don't eat any of it. I just give it away but it's taken so much of my time that I haven't had time to think about anything else. Everyone compliments me about what a great cook I am and they ask me for my secret because I can manage to stay small."

Secondary gain: To keep busy and to receive attention from others and feel valuable.

"I believe that I only get attention from others because I'm small. They want hints and diet tricks too. This makes me feel valuable. I know something they would like to learn."

"I always can blame things on my eating disorder. It's always my reason for why I couldn't do something. Having an eating disoder will always be the answer to why something was not good enough, or why I may have failed in something, or why I'm not living up to my potential or why I'm not in a relationship or have a good job. It's much better to be seen that I could do those things but I have an eating disorder—than the fact that I am really not good enough, lovable enough or smart enough. No one ever questioned why I didn't date in high school. It is because I'm gay and wasn't comfortable. But everyone assumed it was because I'm fat and have an eating disorder."

Secondary gain: Eating disorder identity as protection.

"I always believed that I don't have to try if I have an eating disorder, it takes the pressure off."

"People take care of me and they check on me when I'm not able to do things on my own. It's hard for me to get by. My knees have been in really bad condition and I'm now considered disabled."

Secondary gain: To be taken care of by others.

"I believe that I can't really do things for myself so at least I know that my family won't leave me because I need them."

"When people don't know me, they think I'm strange. I have autism. People don't understand me or the way my brain works. But when I talk about wanting to lose weight, all of a sudden everyone understands me because they want to lose weight too. I can finally relate to others and they can finally understand me."

Secondary gain: To feel normal.

"I don't know how I could be more normal without my eating disorder. I want to be a person with an eating disorder, not a person with autism."

As you can see from the above examples, these individuals are continuing to benefit from having an eating disorder. They are stuck in their belief that they are dependent on their eating disorder. Let's explore your client's beliefs and how they may be benefiting from any secondary gains in the next exercise.

CLIENT EXERCISE: EXPLORING OLD BELIEFS AND SECONDARY GAINS

You might have a love-hate relationship with your eating disorder. While you hate it most of the time and want to be free from it, have you noticed that there's a strange feeling that you may miss it? Having an eating disorder as part of your life for so long can make you feel uncomfortable about letting it go. Did you know that your eating disorder was developed to protect you? You could be still holding on to old beliefs that make you think you still need your eating disorder for protection. That's no longer the case. Let's explore this.

Objective: To create awareness around having an eating disorder identity and how it benefits you.
Directions: Complete the following exercise and discuss with your therapist.

---

1. What are your thoughts, feelings, and beliefs about letting go of your eating disorder?

2. How do you feel about having an eating disorder as a part your identity? In what ways has it benefitted you?

3. What do you feel needs to happen for you to let go of the eating disorder as part of your identity?

Often the old story and patterns that keep an individual stuck is associated with their fears and avoidance about having to deal with the distress in their life. This fear becomes a significant part of their story about who they are and what they are capable of. For example:

Rachel: "Before my eating disorder, I was really different. I was pretty outspoken and I was friendly. I wanted to be around my friends. I wanted to be a part of the activities at school. I didn't even know what self-consciousness was. I only started getting really anxious and fear things as I got older—when my eating disorder developed. I remember feeling really depressed right before my eating disorder started. My mom didn't care that I felt sad all the time. My Mom ignored me and that's when I stopped eating to see if she would care."

Rachel acknowledges the difference before the eating disorder developed. Most people that struggle with disordered eating can recall how they were and the things that they enjoyed before the eating disorder developed. It is important for your client to think about who and how they were before. This helps your client to revisit parts of themselves that they have forgotten existed—the essence of who they were before the eating disorder took over. This will give them a starting point to explore all that is important to them aside from their eating disorder.

CLIENT EXERCISE: IDENTITY BEFORE THE EATING DISORDER

Have you noticed changes in yourself since your eating disorder started? Maybe you used to be a bit more outgoing, or maybe you knew your likes and dislikes. Since you've been struggling with your eating disorder, does it feel like things are more confusing and perhaps you're finding it more difficult to make decisions? Do you feel like you don't even know yourself anymore? If you experience these feelings, know that you're not alone. This is a common struggle. In this exercise, let's explore what it was like before the eating disorder started.

Objective: Bring awareness to what you were like before influences from eating disorder.
Directions: Complete the questions, and discuss with your therapist.

1.   What was your personality like before the eating disorder started?

2.   What were your favorite activities, friends, and/or interests before your eating disorder started?

3.   What was your relationship like with your parents, family members, and/or friends before the eating disorder started?

4.   What challenges were you going through right before the eating disorder started?

5.   Describe who you were as a person before the eating disorder started.

Rachel acknowledged that her mood was low and sad right before her eating disorder started. While depression and anxiety are common underlying factors preceding an eating disorder, many don't make the connection that their eating disorder started as a way to cope with their depression or anxiety. They often confuse the sadness and unsettled feelings associated to the dissatisfaction of their appearance and body image. The things that were important to them get lost, replaced by the distractions of their eating disorder— low self-esteem and their many fears.

When individuals are battling depression and/or generalized anxiety, it is quite common for them to feel helpless and hopeless, that their situation will not improve. They may have tried various medications and its effectiveness changes over time. This can feel discouraging and like an endless battle. Therefore, people that struggle with an eating disorder tend to have difficulty believing that things can change for the better.

This reinforces their story of hopelessness which is further supported by their past negative experiences. They hold on to outdated beliefs about who they are as a person, how their past defines them, or their belief that no amount of effort they put in will ever improve their situation. These beliefs can be rigid—and it can be extremely difficult for them to be willing to apply new behaviors that are needed in order to create lasting change. For example:

> Rachel: *"I'm learning all these new things but honestly, there's a part of me that doubts this will all stick. I've struggled with this for so long. I can't even see how things can change. What if I just can't deal with it? What if I try so hard and still nothing changes? What if I can never fully recover from an eating disorder?"*

Many individuals doubt their ability to fully recover from their eating disorder. Therefore, it is important to address the obstacles and blocks that have thwarted them from believing that lasting eating disorder recovery is obtainable for them. Foundational skill *#9 Changing My Story* is essential to help individuals learn new ways of thinking, behaving, and relating.

Empowering Your Clients to Edit Their Stories

Because depression and anxiety are commonly associated with eating disorder and reinforce their old way of thinking it is important for individuals to be able to make new meaning from their past experiences, ultimately changing their old ineffective story.

Having meaning in your life is a protective factor that counters depression (Marco et al. 2021). and acts as a buffer against negative situations and events (Baquero-Tomás et al. 2023). The three key dimensions of an individual's sense of fulfillment and purpose in living—the motivational force in an authentic and meaningful existence— are coherence, purpose, and significance. When individuals are struggling with depression, an eating disorder, and a sense of who they are, through social influence, they often misinterpret and search for significance, purpose and connection by obtaining the accepted social standard ideal in their physical appearance. They are derailed from their search for real meaning and what their soul is yearning for (Landau 2018).

They need to connect to a life that matters and that is worth living for. This is usually experienced as freedom, responsibility and self-determination, fulfilment of life goals, having a positive view on life, of the future, and self-realization. Most of these are absent from the lives of people who struggle with recurrent depression and eating disorders. When these are not achieved, as observed in our clients, they are left frustrated, feeling hopeless, having doubts, and perceive a lack of control over their lives with no sense of direction or goals. Their perceived meaning of life is strongly correlated to their happiness (Sameer et al. 2023).

While there isn't an innate human need for meaning, perceived meaning in life affects people's satisfaction overall. This is observed more obviously when one is miserable and questions their life. People who are sorrowful are more aware of the lack of meaning in their life and can attribute their dissatisfaction to not having a purpose, meaning, or significance. Therefore, it is important for individuals who are recovering from their eating disorder to cultivate meaning in their lives, enabling them to change their old beliefs about their current and future situation (Marco et al. 2019.). This is essential to human functioning—and the benefits include a sense of wellbeing, reduced suicidal ideation, and lower depression and anxiety (Marco et al. 2020.).

Let's explore this with your client. Often individuals struggle with identifying what's important to them. In the next exercise, let's use a "book" as a metaphor to help your client understand that they have more control in their life than they realize. This book represents your client's "life story". This will help your client to identify areas that are significant for them and recognize that they have the power to edit and change their story. This is a valuable tool that your client will be able to practice whenever they feel stuck or when they notice an "old story" replaying. They have the power to edit or change their story at any time.

For example, let's take a look at Rachel.

Rachel: "In chapter one of my life story, my mom basically chose where I lived and the school I attended. But I guess when I look at the middle chapters (that's where I am now), I have a few people in my life that are not supportive. I have an ex-boyfriend who is toxic but still a part of my life. I feel like I keep using my eating disorder to deal with him. This is why I feel like nothing will ever change for me because—he will never change. Things will never be better."

In Rachel's current story, she believes that her boyfriend will never change. Rachel continually forgets that she is the author of her story and that she has the power to change things. However, she has accepted that her ex-boyfriend continues to treat her negatively—and believes that her life cannot get better because of this. In this situation she has an external locus of control, believing that the power to change things is in the hands of her ex-boyfriend. However, Rachel can edit and change her story by creating boundaries with her ex-boyfriend or since she is the author of her life story, she can write this ex-boyfriend character out of her story. She no longer has to accept being treated negatively.

Let's try this exercise with your client.

CLIENT EXERCISE: SHAPING MY LIFE STORY

Have you ever imagined what it would be like if you had a magic wand? You may have wanted a magic wand to give you what you want in your life, and to take away the things that you don't like. However, what if instead of a magic wand, you had a magic pen? This magic pen gives you the power to edit and make changes in your life story. If you had the opportunity to be the author of your own life story what edits and changes would you make? Let's find out.

Objective: Recognize that you have the power to edit and to make changes necessary for a meaningful life story and to identify what is important and meaningful for you.

What you will need:

- Journal book.
- Pen.
- Quiet room.
- 60–75 minutes.

Directions: Find a comfortable place to sit where you will be undisturbed for at least an hour. Grab your journal and favorite pen, and respond to the writing prompts. Afterward, complete the reflection questions worksheet.

---

1. Close your eyes and imagine the first chapters in your life: your first years of life up until adolescence. You didn't get to make decisions about where you would live, who your parents were, or what school you attended etc. You didn't get to choose your family members or relatives. These chapters have already been written for you.
2. Now imagine the next chapters in your life. You are an adult, and you get to use your magic pen. Now close your eyes and think about the questions below which will help you to start thinking about what you find important. You may add your own questions. Then write the responses in your journal.

- Who are the characters in your current chapter?
- What is the theme in your current chapter?
- What would you like to edit or change in your current story?
- Who are the most supportive characters? Who are the least supportive?
- What would you like to see happen in your current story?
- What is most important for you in your story?
- What do you wish for yourself in your current story? How could you make that happen?
- If there were no obstacles, blocks or resistance, what would you want for yourself in your wildest dreams (that doesn't relate to body image or eating disorder thoughts)?

3. After you have written about what is happening in your current chapter, close your eyes and imagine the last chapter of your story. You are in the future, in the last chapter of your life. What is important to you at that point in your life? What have you done, achieved, accomplished, or completed? How would you want others to remember you? Think about these questions and write them in your journal.

- Who are the characters in your last chapter?
- What do you want your last chapter theme to be about?
- How would you like to feel in your last chapter in your story?
- What is important to you in your last chapter of your book?
- Who are the characters that are most important to you?
- How would you like to be remembered by others?
- What legacy would you like to leave behind?
- What are the three things that you are most proud of in your last chapter?
- What was most meaningful to as you reflect back on your life?
- Are there anything you wished you would have done in your last chapter of your life?

4. Finally, re-read your answers to the previous questions. Then close your eyes and think about what you wrote about your last chapter. Now, imagine the string of chapters that will come between your current chapter and the last one. What needs to happen in your current chapter and the ones that follow to result in what you recorded in the last chapter? In other words, what needs to happen in your life now to reach your goals? Answer the following questions in your journal.

- What changes can you make now?
- Who are the characters that can support you in your last chapter? Who are the characters that most likely will become obstacles?
- How can you write these characters out of your story?
- How can you identify new supportive characters for your story?
- What is important to you?
- What edits and changes do you need to make now in your current story in order to support your last chapter?
- Identify your current obstacles, resistances, and blocks in your story. How do you write these obstacles, resistances and blocks out of your story?

Reflection Questions

1. What did you notice about your thoughts, feelings, and behaviors when completing the exercise?

2. How does it feel to be able to make edits and changes in your story?

3. Identify any challenges that you experienced when completing the exercise.

4. What did you learn about yourself through this process?

5. What did you find most important for you with this process?

Occasionally when doing this exercise, individuals will have difficulty with dichotomous thinking. They get stuck thinking about the first chapters of their lives during which they had no control over the decisions that were made for them. Therefore, it is important to address the first few chapters of the individuals' lives by helping them to view their past with meaning. This is done by a process called *simulation*, see below.

Identifying Meaning, Purpose, and Significance

Simulation involves mentally transcending the "here and now." Also known as *self-projection*, it's a technique that allows individuals to psychologically involve themselves in a different time, place, perspective, and to experience a hypothetical reality (Waytz et al. 2015). This process enables individuals to call forth another experience other than their own.

Studies support the idea that specific forms of simulation are related to meaning in life for example, both *retrospection* and *prospection* appear to enhance meaning (Waytz et al. 2015). This is an important concept because people who struggle with disordered eating have difficulty with consciousness and awareness. Simulation requires consciousness. For example, nostalgia, the process of sentimentally reflecting on past events, has been shown to increase perceived meaning in life. Individuals are able to reflect about the past and perceive those events differently than they did while they were actually experiencing. Instead of focusing on negative memories and past trauma, individuals can take a look back on their lives and identify experiences that they valued, such as family time, experiencing life, and being okay with who they were before their disordered eating struggles. This includes everyday activities such as foods they enjoyed, or routine life experiences with friends and family such as wardrobe shopping or gatherings. For example:

> Rachel: "I can think back about my life, and I can honestly say that it wasn't all bad. Yes, I had some really difficult times, but I do think about how much fun I had with friends before the eating problems got really bad. It does make me think about what's really important to me."

It is essential that your client can reflect back on their lives and identify situations that felt enjoyable, positive, and/or sentimental. While they may have been challenging, memories of these times will show them the deeper meaning behind the experience and they will be able to recognize their own growth. This eventually allows them to edit their life story. In the next exercise, your client will explore meaning from their past experiences. This can be a corrective experience as they make new meaning from old stories that have been obstacles.

CLIENT WORKSHEET: NOSTALGIC MEANING MAKING

Do you remember childhood summers, the neighborhood kids, or your favorite games? Or perhaps, you have a memory of your favorite pet growing up, or your favorite teacher? While positive memories are easily overlooked often by hardships in your life, it is important to remember that the positives as well as the hardships make up who you are today.

Objective: Practicing retrospection to create meaning from past experiences.
Directions: Complete the worksheet and discuss with your therapist.

1. What was your favorite food, color, and television show growing up?

2. Describe your best friends and or favorite teachers. What memories do you have of them?

3. Describe the most memorable time spent with an important figure in your life growing up.

4. Describe your favorite places where you felt peaceful and carefree.

5. Describe a time where you were most proud of yourself.

6. Describe something that was important to you growing up.

Another form of simulation is known as *counterfactual thinking*. This is reimagining past events, expanding them, and giving them a hypothetical spin (Waytz et al. 2015). to enhance perceptions about the situation, which helps individuals to make meaning from those events. For example, in counterfactual thinking, our clients can imagine what their younger years would have been like if they didn't have an eating disorder, or what might have happened if they'd gone on that date in high school. This helps individuals gain clarity about some of their dreams, passions, and values.

Often people who struggle with eating experience hypersensitivity in their reactions to specific situations. This is a challenge for them and they may get caught up in the emotion, causing them to experience *emotional flooding*. Therefore, learning to self-distance, mentally step outside of themselves, or learn to adopt a third-person perspective on personal events and past situations can help them to derive meaning from these situations using a less emotional response. This enables them to seek a deeper meaning rather than focusing on the negative experience and reliving the emotional pain.

In the next exercise, your client will practice taking a step back and reviewing their past from a distant perspective to find the deeper meanings and lessons of growth from each experience.

CLIENT WORKSHEET: TAKING A STEP BACK

Have you ever experienced something that seemed terrible in the moment only to look back at it later and realize it wasn't so bad? When you reflect on a distressing event after time has passed, you might conclude that it was actually a blessing in disguise. Perhaps it if weren't for that situation something else may not have happened. With hindsight, you can look at your life from various perspectives and often find new meaning in past situations. Let's practice stepping back and looking at past situations that were challenging.

Objective: To find new meaning in past situations by taking a step back and looking at it from a different perspective.

Directions: Complete the following questions and discuss with your therapist.

1. Describe a situation that you wished you had handled differently. How do you wish you had the situation?

2. Describe a situation that still bothers you today. If you were the observer of this situation, what would you have done?

3. Describe a past situation that felt difficult when going through it, but perceive differently today.

4. Describe an experience that you feel contributes to you positively today.

5. How do you feel your past experiences helped you grow?

Looking to Future Legacies and Goals

Another way that individuals can initiate meaning in their life is by thinking positively about their future. When our clients are in eating disorder treatment they often experience anxiety when they think about the future because they are constantly ruminating about future fears. However, once they are able to manage their anxiety and have the foundational skills to deal with their fears it is important for them to think about their dreams, passions, and goals. This helps them to create meaning, significance, and purpose in their life. For example:

> Rachel: "Whenever I think about the future, it brings up a lot of anxiety for me. I just think about how scary things will be. Therefore, I always avoided thinking about the future. I have never thought about what I want for my future. I just never really thought that I had the power to create something for myself."

This is common for individuals who struggle with eating. Many have never thought about possibilities for their future. In fact, many haven't imagined that they would still be alive after a certain age and therefore have never really thought about what they want for their future. It is necessary for your clients to explore what they want for their future, and to identify what is important for them so they can start to visualize life outside an eating disorder.

CLIENT WORKSHEET: FINDING SIGNIFICANCE, MEANING, AND PURPOSE

Do you remember role playing as a child? Perhaps, you imagined yourself as a parent, or a doctor, or a teacher. Your imagination ran wild, free from the limitations that would be later imposed by parents, siblings, and others. Imagine, being that child again—filled with wonder and inspiration. Going back to that time, what were some things that you couldn't wait to do? What were things that woke your curiosity and fed your creativity? Let's explore areas today that help you to feel alive—and that you want to see more of in your life.

Objective: To tap into the excitement and creativity that lives inside of you.

Directions: Complete the questions in the worksheet and discuss with your therapist.

---

1. As a child, what did you want to be when you grew up?

2. What did you naturally gravitate towards to as a child?

3. What brought excitement and fulfilment to you?

4. What compliments or positive feedback did others give you?

5. What were your strengths that others have pointed out to you?

6. What do you feel your strengths are today?

7. What brings excitement and fulfilment to you today?

8. Identify three goals that you would like to complete within the next 12 months. Describe your plan to reach these goals.

People who have suffered from an eating disorder for many years may find it incredibly challenging to adopt a different perspective. While these previous exercises are important for your client to explore, for some individuals their rigid thinking and inflexibility commonly become obstacles. Therefore, if you notice that your clients are experiencing difficulty with the retrospection and prospection exercises or worksheets, the following tools can help. These tools are meant to support your client in their flexibility and in changing their behaviors. Using these tools will enable your client to be open to new ideas, new behavioral changes, and open to a new story.

Using Tools and Activities that Support a New Story

Tools that can help support your client in their ability to change their story can be practiced daily to help with inflexibility, rigid thoughts, and behaviors. Often, your clients have been doing the same thing for a long period of time. This has become safe and comfortable for them—even when it's no longer benefitting them or is keeping them from growing.

Eating disorders often involve experiences of anxiety and fear and to this end exposure-based intervention can improve treatment for these complicated symptoms and disorders (Schaumberg et al. 2020). Therefore, it is important for your clients to practice the following tools to be help cultivate foundational skill #9 *Changing My Story*.

Psychological Flexibility

This can be cultivated by engaging in new things, such as learning a new language or learning to play a new instrument. Your clients can look for new opportunities such as meeting new people in a class, or doing something out of the ordinary. Furthermore, flexibility can be practiced by expanding their horizons and making their world bigger. They can join a group, a class, or volunteer in a community program.

If those ideas feel overwhelming for your client they can start with something they already do normally, only they have to do it a little differently. For example, if they drive the same route every day, or use the same dish, pillow, or choose the same colors to wear, your client will have to do something different, maybe eating out of a different dish every day, using different utensils, choosing a different pillow, or taking the long way to work. Changing things up for your client helps them with psychological flexibility.

It is common for individuals who struggle with disordered eating to do the same things over and over because it feels safe and comfortable for them. Changing the dish and or asking them to use a different utensil can make them feel uneasy. Therefore, while these changes appear small, it will still benefit them over time.

ANCHORING

Events and situations can remind your client of the past and can trigger an old story. For example, smelling glue might take your client back to an experience as a child, or listening to an old song could take them back to their first heart break. These situations can bring up insecurities, fears, and worries. Therefore, your client needs to create new anchors to remind them that they are no longer the scared little child, or insecure teen. In anchoring, your client will choose a positive object that they can conveniently carry with them. For example, Rachel wore a rubber bracelet.

> Rachel: *"Okay, I have to say this anchoring thing does work. I wear this rubber bracelet, and when I feel triggered about something, I immediately remove the bracelet and put it on my other wrist. This is a reminder that I am an adult and I am no longer a scared child. I've been doing this for a few weeks now, and noticed I no longer feel stuck."*

Resourcing Techniques

In resourcing, your client will imagine whatever distress they are experiencing played out on a movie screen. They will describe what they see. They will imagine all their discomforts and when the images are really disturbing they can freeze the screen. They will then imagine a tiny bubble in the corner of their screen. Then they will imagine popping the bubble and having the liquid ooze out all over the screen. The entire screen is then covered with the positive image. Finally, your client will imagine the bubble bursting and their positive image will take over the screen. They will then continue to imagine that they have the power to change the image to whatever image they find helpful for them.

Another option that your client can use for resourcing is to draw an image of their uncomfortable story. Then using another piece of paper, your client will draw the opposite story and focus on what they want to happen instead. They are then asked to only think about what they want to happen and how explore how they can make that happen.

The "remote control" resource is a tool that your client can use to change the channel any time something disturbing comes on. Your client will notice their thoughts and when they notice something disturbing they can change the channel to something that is calming instead.

Your client has the power to focus on the disturbing images by slowing the images down, pausing, or even zooming in on certain images. When they are ready to change the channel, they can do it at any time. You can then ask "What would you like see instead?" Instruct your client to draw an image that helps them feel secure and ask them to post it somewhere in their home that can act as a reminder that their story is on edit.

These tools are important and helpful for your clients when their old story starts to sneak up on them. These coping tools help your client to feel in control and when they can effectively utilize these tools it changes their thinking that things will never get better. This leads to more open, flexible thinking and builds their confidence becuase the very act of utilizing these tools is already a change in their story.

It is important for your clients to identify what they want to see in their lives. However, if this is something your client has never practiced, they will have some challenges to start with. However, like everything else, with practice, they will be able to come up with a long list of things that are significant and meaningful for them. This list will give them a starting place to establish and identify their goals.

CLIENT EXERCISE: WHAT DO YOU WANT IN YOUR LIFE?

You may not have given your wants much thought lately. But let's change that by bringing focus to the things you want to see in your life. The more time you spend thinking about these things, the more likely you are act on opportunities to make them a tangible part of your life.

Objective: Bring awareness to what you want to see in your life
Directions:

1. Create a long list of everything that you want: Material, spiritual, psychological.
2. Then meditate on the list for a while. Did you include everything? What are your biggest wants or needs?
3. Then distill the list to the ten most important things that you want.
4. Every day, at least once a day, but three times is even better, look at the list. You can glance at the list on your phone or just close your eyes and mentally bring it to mind. Do this for several weeks.
5. You don't need tell anyone about your list. But you can discuss with your therapist.

Make a list of everything you want: Material, spiritual, psychological.

Make a list of the top ten things you want in your life.

Establishing Connections

Finally, a significant part of eating disorder recovery is having a sense of connection. The lack of connection keeps your client feeling isolated and dependent on their eating disorder. However, meaningful connection and meaningful relationships are supportive and a corrective experience to replace their lack of connection growing up (Linville et al. 2012).

CLIENT EXERCISE: SOCIAL CONNECTION

Social connection is an important aspect of recovery from your eating disorder. A big part of successful eating disorder recovery is practicing these skills while still in therapy with your therapist. This allows you to have support while transitioning—to be able to share and work through any challenges that may surface.

Objective: Identify and apply opportunities for social connections
Directions: Identify opportunities for social connections and participate in the events. Discuss with your therapist.

1. Identify any groups or organizations that you are willing to be a part of.

2. Identify any friendships or relationships you would like to explore.

3. Identify any supportive people, groups, community members that you can reach out to.

4. Identify your social connection goals. Describe three goals that you would like to reach.

5. What is your plan to obtain the three social connection goals?

Being a part of a group, community, or organization can help your client fulfill new opportunities, meet new people, have new experiences, and grow exponentially. This will give your client the opportunity to learn more about themselves, and to identify their values, passions, and pursuits.

Community connection gives your client a place to practice their psychosocial functioning skills. Further, research suggests community connection, being a part of the community, is an indicator for lasting eating disorder recovery. Therefore, before terminating your client's treatment, and as an important part of their discharge plan, it is essential that your client is connected to a group, community, or organization that they find meaningful.

Bibliography

Baquero-Tomás, M., Grau, M. D., Moliner, A. R., & Sanchis-Sanchis, A. (2023). Meaning in life as a protective factor against depression. *Frontiers in Psychology*, *14*, 1180082. https://doi.org/10.3389/fpsyg.2023.1180082.

Ferrier-Auerbach, A. G., & Martens, M. P. (2009). Perceived incompetence moderates the relationship between maladaptive perfectionism and disordered eating. *Eating Disorders*, *17*(4), 333–344. DOI: 10.1080/10640260902991244.

Gerber, S., & Folta, S. C. (2022). You Are What You Eat... But Do You Eat What You Are? The Role of Identity in Eating Behaviors–A Scoping Review. *Nutrients, 14*(17), 3456. DOI: 10.3390/nu14173456.

Ison, J., & Kent, S. Social identity in eating disorders. *European Eating Disorder Review, 18*(6), 475–485. DOI: 10.1002/erv.1001.

Landau, M. J. (2018). Using Metaphor to Find Meaning in Life. *Review of General Psychology: Journal of Division 1 of the American Psychological Association, 22*(1), 62–72. https://doi.org/10.1037/gpr0000105.

Linville, D., Brown, T., Sturm, K., & McDougal, T. (2012). Eating disorders and social support: perspectives of recovered individuals. *Eating Disorders, 20*(3), 216–231.

Marco, J. H., Cañabate, M., & Pérez, S. (2019). Meaning in life is associated with the psychopathology of eating disorders: differences depending on the diagnosis. *Eating Disorders, 27*(6), 550–564. DOI: 10.1080/10640266.2018.1560852.

Marco, J. H., Cañabate, M., Llorca, G., & Pérez, S. (2020). Meaning in life moderates hopelessness, suicide ideation, and borderline psychopathology in participants with eating disorders: A longitudinal study. *Clinical Psychology & Psychotherapy, 27*(2), 146–158. https://doi.org/10.1002/cpp.2414.

Marco, J. H. et al. (2021). Meaning in Life Mediates Between Emotional Deregulation and Eating Disorders Psychopathology: A Research From the Meaning-Making Model of Eating Disorders. *Frontiers in Psychology, 12*, 635742. https://doi.org/10.3389/fpsyg.2021.635742.

McNamara, N, & Parsons,. H. (2016). "Everyone here wants everyone else to get better": The role of social identity in eating disorder recovery. *British Journal of Social Psychology, 55*(4), 662–680. DOI: 10.1111/bjso.12161.

Sameer, Y., Eid, Y., & Veenhoven, R. (2023). Perceived meaning of life and satisfaction with life: A research synthesis using an online finding archive. *Frontiers in Psychology, 13*, 957235. https://doi.org/10.3389/fpsyg.2022.957235.

Schaumberg, K. et al. (2021). Conceptualizing eating disorder psychopathology using an anxiety disorders framework: Evidence and implications for exposure-based clinical research. *Clinical Psychology Review, 83*, 101952. https://doi.org/10.1016/j.cpr.2020.101952.

Waytz, A., Hershfield, H. E., & Tamir, D. I. (2015). Mental simulation and meaning in life. *Journal of Personality and Social Psychology, 108*(2), 336–355. https://doi.org/10.1037/a0038322.

Epilogue

As busy clinicians, we are always seeking more efficient ways of completing clinical paperwork. We can all relate to easily falling behind in our treatment plan documentation, clinical notes, and just charting in general.

The nine foundational skills for eating disorder recovery were developed with the busy clinician in mind. They make it easy to identify the skills their clients need to target. They become a clinical shorthand when completing clinical notes. Below are parts of sample forms, such as a treatment plan, SOAP (Subjective, Objective, Assessment and Plan) note, and a discharge plan that demonstrates how therapists can easily document the foundational skills in their notes. This makes charting quicker and more efficient because each foundational skill identified is part of the treatment plan and will identify the challenges that the client is facing. These notes can then be added to the discharge summaries with the dates completed.

Rachel's Sample Treatment Plan: Sessions 1–5

This is an example of part of Rachel's treatment plan that was completed after her first intake appointment.

Treatment Goal #1	Intervention/Modality	Specific Skills to Practice
Reduce binge eating episodes	*Foundational skill #1 Establishing a Mind-Body Connection*	*Rachel will practice tuning into her body and rating her hunger cues before eating and when she is finished eating.*
	Foundational skill #2 Uncovering the Meaning Behind Food and Eating	*Rachel will journal feelings and practice decoding food if not physically hungry.*

Treatment Goal #2	Intervention /Modality	Specific Skills to Practice
Improve Negative Mood	*Foundational skill #3 Quieting Negative Thoughts*	*Rachel will practice neutralizing her thoughts.*
		Rachel will take mindful walks in nature daily after work.

DOI: 10.4324/9781032651408-18

Clinician Tool: Treatment Plan

Treatment Goal #1	Intervention/Modality	Specific Skills to Practice

Treatment Goal #2	Intervention /Modality	Specific Skills to Practice

Rachel's Sample SOAP Note: Session #3

This is an example of part of a clinical SOAP note that was completed in session 3 with Rachel.

Subjective:

"I binged last night. I couldn't stop eating. It started after getting off the phone with my mom. She said some things that were really hurtful to me. I know it's not the right way to deal with it but I was so angry."

Objective:

Rachel was present and alert. She was able to track her thoughts while in session and made good eye contact.

Assessment:

Rachel has difficulty with skills #6, #7, and #8.

She struggles with the relationship with her mother and understanding her mother's perspective. She is also struggling with tolerating emotional triggers and in setting appropriate boundaries with her mother.

Plan:

Rachel will practice skills from #6, #7, and # 8.

Rachel will explore her needs in session for skill #6, and #7.

She will practice putting words to what she is feeling and will practice writing it out and practice the assertiveness formula for follow up.

Next session: in a week.

Clinician Tool: SOAP note

Subjective:
Objective:
Assessment:
Plan:

Rachel's Sample Discharge Plan

This is a part of a discharge plan that was completed a week before Rachel was discharged. The completion dates will obviously vary. Rachel did terminate therapy because she completed all treatment goals.

Problem: Binge Eating Disorder

Long Term Goal	Intervention	Completed Date	Follow up/ Notes
Reduce Binge Eating to 0– 1x weekly.	_Foundational skills #1 & 2._	_Completed on 2/2/2023_	_Rachel can easily differentiate emotional vs physical hunger. She can utilize alternative strategies when the urge arises._
Reduce negative mood by using adaptive coping strategies	_Foundational skills #3 & 4._	_Completed on 2/2/2023_	_Rachel can practice skills to reduce negative thoughts._
Self- acceptance by showing herself kindness and self-compassion	_Foundational skills #4, 5, 6._	_Completed on 2/2/2023_	_Rachel can verbalize positive aspects about herself and exhibits self-compassion and self-acceptance by practicing kind behaviors towards herself._
Functioning in a meaningful job	_Foundational skills #7,8, 9_	_Completed on 2/2/2023_	_Rachel will be starting her new job as coordinator at the local animal shelter._
Establish social support/ connection and being a part of a group or organization at least 3x a week.	_Foundational skills #7, 8, 9_	_Completed 2/2/2023_	_Rachel has been a part of the local animal shelter for over a year. She is the organizer of event and is also employed there. She has connections with volunteers, co-workers and is part of the community._

Clinician Tool: Discharge Plan

Long Term Goal	Intervention	Completed Date	Follow up/ Notes

Long Term Goal	Intervention	Completed Date	Follow up/ Notes

Farewell Message

I sincerely hope that you have found this book helpful. My intention was to teach my readers how to effectively approach such an intimidating and complex disorder. My wish for you is that you will find the confidence in working with this population—and that you will experience great satisfaction knowing that you have helped your clients overcome, and live a life free from, their eating disorder.

Index

Note: **Bold** page numbers indicate tables, *italic* numbers indicate figures.

Printed in the United States
by Baker & Taylor Publisher Services